PROJECT PLANNING *and* MANAGEMENT

A GUIDE FOR CNLs, DNPs, AND NURSE EXECUTIVES

Edited by

James L. Harris, DSN, APRN-BC, MBA, CNL, FAAN
Consultant
Washington, DC

Linda Roussel, DSN, RN, NEA-BC, CNL
Professor and Coordinator
Executive Nurse and Clinical Nurse Leader Programs
University of South Alabama
College of Nursing
Mobile, Alabama

Sandra E. Walters, DNP, RN
Department of Veterans Affairs
Tennessee Valley Healthcare System
Nashville, Tennessee

Catherine Dearman, PhD, RN
Professor and Associate Dean
Research and Development
University of South Alabama
College of Nursing
Mobile, Alabama

D0556454

JONES & BARTLETT
LEARNING

World Headquarters

Jones & Bartlett Learning
40 Tall Pine Drive
Sudbury, MA 01776
978-443-5000
info@jblearning.com
www.jblearning.com

Jones & Bartlett Learning
Canada
6339 Ormindale Way
Mississauga, Ontario L5V 1J2
Canada

Jones & Bartlett Learning
International
Barb House, Barb Mews
London W6 7PA
United Kingdom

Jones & Bartlett Learning books and products are available through most bookstores and online booksellers. To contact Jones & Bartlett Learning directly, call 800-832-0034, fax 978-443-8000, or visit our website, www.jblearning.com.

Substantial discounts on bulk quantities of Jones & Bartlett Learning publications are available to corporations, professional associations, and other qualified organizations. For details and specific discount information, contact the special sales department at Jones & Bartlett Learning via the above contact information or send an email to specialsales@jblearning.com.

The authors, editor, and publisher have made every effort to provide accurate information. However, they are not responsible for errors, omissions, or for any outcomes related to the use of the contents of this book and take no responsibility for the use of the products and procedures described. Treatments and side effects described in this book may not be applicable to all people; likewise, some people may require a dose or experience a side effect that is not described herein. Drugs and medical devices are discussed that may have limited availability controlled by the Food and Drug Administration (FDA) for use only in a research study or clinical trial. Research, clinical practice, and government regulations often change the accepted standard in this field. When consideration is being given to use of any drug in the clinical setting, the health care provider or reader is responsible for determining FDA status of the drug, reading the package insert, and reviewing prescribing information for the most up-to-date recommendations on dose, precautions, and contraindications, and determining the appropriate usage for the product. This is especially important in the case of drugs that are new or seldom used.

Production Credits
Publisher: Kevin Sullivan
Acquisitions Editor: Amy Sibley
Associate Editor: Patricia Donnelly
Editorial Assistant: Rachel Shuster
Associate Production Editor: Katie Spiegel
Associate Marketing Manager: Katie Hennessy
V.P., Manufacturing and Inventory
  Control: Therese Connell
Composition: diacriTech
Cover Design: Scott Moden
Cover Image: © Bocos Benedict/ShutterStock, Inc.
Printing and Binding: Malloy, Inc.
Cover Printing: Malloy, Inc.

Library of Congress Cataloging-in-Publication Data
Project planning and management : a guide for CNLs, DNPs, and nurse executives / James L. Harris . . . [et al.].
    p. ; cm.
Includes bibliographical references and index.
ISBN 978-0-7637-8586-4 (pbk.)
1. Nursing services—Administration. 2. Project management. I. Harris, James L. (James Leonard), 1956–
[DNLM: 1. Nursing—organization & administration. 2. Nursing Assessment—methods. 3. Nursing Research—methods. 4. Planning Techniques. 5. Program Development. WY 105 P9647 2011]
RT89.P765 2011
610.73068—dc22

                    2010017896

6048
Printed in the United States of America
14 13 12 11 10   10 9 8 7 6 5 4 3 2 1

CONTENTS

CHAPTER TWELVE
Anna C. Alt-White and Maryann F. Pranulis

CHAPTER THIRTEEN

CHAPTER FOURTEEN

PREFACE

The dynamic and constantly evolving changes in the healthcare environment require individuals to forge ahead with innovative planning and solutions. In an era of technology-driven business decisions, the ability of nurses to maintain the competitive edge can be enhanced by project management skills. From project idea to implementation, skill sets that capitalize on project management and information technology are requisite for success. As e-nursing, telehealth, and telemedicine continue to revolutionize how nurses interact with patients, families, and other team members, nursing is in a unique position to develop projects and programs that meet the challenges inherent in the needs of a global society.

This textbook is a composite of strategies, techniques, and exemplars that guide the development, implementation, and evaluation of projects and programs that can be sustained over time. We are grateful to the ongoing actions of project developers, managers, and educators who partner daily to advance nursing, improving the quality and safety of the patient care experience.

Thank you,

James L. Harris, Linda Roussel,

Sandra E. Walters, and Catherine Dearman

ACKNOWLEDGMENTS

My colleagues and I acknowledge each of the contributors to this textbook and the educators and mentors who have guided our careers. Vision, determination, persistence, and an open mind are hallmarks for successful project planning and program management. To our friends and families who supported this endeavor, we treasure your ongoing support and thank you. Without your unwavering commitment to professional development, this work would not have been possible. For this we are grateful.

CONTRIBUTORS

Anna C. Alt-White, PhD, RN
Director, Research and Academic Programs
Department of Veterans Affairs
Washington, DC

Mark Balch, MHA
Health Systems Specialist
Department of Veterans Affairs
Washington, DC

Amy Beard, MSN, RN
Administrative Director
Women's Services at Brookwood Medical Center
Birmingham, Alabama

Murielle S. Beene, MS, PPH, BBA, RN-BC, PMP
Chief Informatics Officer
Department of Veterans Affairs
Washington, DC

Alan Bernstein, MS, RN
Director, Career Development and Workforce Management
Department of Veterans Affairs
Washington, DC

Michael R. Bleich, PhD, RN, FAAN
Dean and Dr. Carol A Lindeman Distinguished Professor
Oregon Health and Science University
School of Nursing
Portland, Oregon

Henri Brown, DNP, RN
Assistant Professor
University of South Alabama
College of Nursing
Mobile, Alabama

Clista Clanton, MSLS
Education Coordinator
Baugh Biomedical Library
University of South Alabama
Mobile, Alabama

Bonny Collins, MPA, PA-C
Director, Informatics
Department of Veterans Affairs
Washington, DC

Sharon Cusanza, MSN, RN, CPHQ
Special Projects Director
Ochsner Foundation Hospital
Jefferson, Louisiana

Debra Davis, DSN, RN
Professor and Dean
University of South Alabama
College of Nursing
Mobile, Alabama

Catherine Dearman, PhD, RN
Professor and Associate Dean
Research and Development
University of South Alabama
College of Nursing
Mobile, Alabama

Valorie Dearmon, DNP, RN
University of South Alabama
College of Nursing
Mobile, Alabama

Alicia Drew, MSN, RN, CNL
Director of Clinical Operations
University of Oklahoma College of Nursing
Oklahoma City, Oklahoma

Gregory S. Eagerton, DNP, RN, NEA-BC
Associate Director for Patient/Nursing Service
VA Medical Center
Birmingham, Alabama

Mary Geary, PhD, RN
Vice President, Safety
Mobile Infirmary Systems
Mobile, Alabama

Drew Glazner, MSN, RN
Staff Development
University of South Alabama Medical Center
Mobile, Alabama

Mimi Haberfelde, MS, RN
Nursing Informatics Specialist
Department of Veterans Affairs
San Francisco, California

Joyce A. Hahn, PhD, APRN, NEA-BC
Assistant Dean, Master's Division
School of Nursing
George Mason University
Fairfax, Virginia

James L. Harris, DSN, APRN-BC, MBA, CNL, FAAN
Consultant
Washington, DC

Reji John, MBA, MHA, FACHE
Health Systems Specialist
Department of Veterans Affairs
Washington, DC

Cynthia R. King, PhD, RN, NP
Faculty
Queens University of Charlotte
Charlotte, North Carolina

Robin Lawson, DNP, RN, CRNP
University of South Alabama
College of Nursing
Mobile, Alabama

Alicia Levin, MS, RN
Nursing Informatics Specialist
Department of Veterans Affairs
San Francisco, California

Paula Miller, MSN, RN, CNL
Department of Veterans Affairs
Augusta, Georgia

Marie Eileen Onieal, PhD, MMHS, RN, CPNP, FAANP
Graduate Program Director, Doctorate of Nursing Practice
Rocky Mountain University of Health Professions
Provo, Utah

Karen M. Ott, MSN, RN
Clinical Executive
Department of Veterans Affairs
Washington, DC

Sandra L. Pennington, PhD, RN
Academic Dean
Rocky Mountain University of Health Professions
Provo, Utah

Pam Pickett, MSN, RN
Nursing Informatics Specialist
Department of Veterans Affairs
White River Junction, Vermont

Becky Pomrenke, MSN, RN, CNL
University of South Alabama
College of Nursing
Mobile, Alabama

Maryann F. Pranulis, DNSc
Principal Consultant
M. F. Pranulis & Associates
Frederick, Maryland

Carol J. Radcliffe, DNP, RN, CNOR, FACHE
Vice President, Patient Care Services
St. Vincent's East
Birmingham, Alabama

Kerrian Reynolds, MPH
Health Systems Specialist
Department of Veterans Affairs
Washington, DC

Cathy Rick, RN, NEA-BC, FACHE, FAAN
Chief Nursing Officer
Department of Veterans Affairs
Washington, DC

Linda Roussel, DSN, RN, NEA-BC, CNL
Professor and Coordinator
Executive Nurse and Clinical Nurse Leader Programs
University of South Alabama
College of Nursing
Mobile, Alabama

Traci Solt, MSN, RN
Acting Director, Education
VA Gulf Coast Veterans Healthcare System
Biloxi, Mississippi

Patricia L. Thomas, PhD, RN, NEA-BC
Associate Professor
McAutry School of Nursing
College of Health Professions
University of Detroit-Michigan
Detroit, Michigan

Susan Thomas, MSN, RN, CNL
CCU Staff/Charge Nurse
Mobile Infirmary Medical Center
Infirmary Health System
Mobile, Alabama

Julie Tragott, MSN, RN
Manager, Clinical Risk Operations
Children's Healthcare of Atlanta
Atlanta, Georgia

Sandra E. Walters, DNP, RN
Department of Veterans Affairs
Tennessee Valley Healthcare System
Nashville, Tennessee

Lonnie K. Williams, MSN, RN
Educator
Nashville, Tennessee

ONE

From Project Planning to Program Management

■ James L. Harris and Linda Roussel

■ **Learning Objectives**

1. Compare and contrast project planning with program management.
2. Identify antecedents and empirical referents related to project planning and program management.
3. Describe projects as a means of achieving an organization's strategic plan.
4. Explore processes to measure meaningful project outcomes in support of a program.

> "Government is not reason, it is not eloquence—it is a force! Like fire, it is a dangerous servant and a fearful master; never for a moment should it be left to irresponsible action."
>
> —George Washington

Key Terms

Evaluation

Innovation

Organizational readiness

Program management

Project planning

Stakeholders

Strategic planning

Value

Roles

Advocate

Communicator

Decision maker

Designer

Educator

Integrator

Leader

Risk anticipator

Professional Values

Altruism

Evidence-based practice

Integrity

Patient-centric care

Quality

Core Competencies

Appreciative inquiry

Assessment

Communication

Coordination

Critical thinking

Design

Emotional intelligence

Health promotion

Information

Interpersonal influence

Leadership

Management

Resource management

Risk reduction

Systems thinking

Technology

Introduction

What a profound quotation by one of our founding fathers and the first president of the United States. The statement has a familiar ring when one considers its relevance to planning projects, implementing them, and managing programs amid the numerous and complex challenges facing healthcare organizations and systems. Planning and implementing projects require a rigorous application of appreciative inquiry, critical and creative thinking, and **strategic planning** and analysis. The development of a sound business case identifying a valid need and opportunities for sustainable outcomes are requisite for improvement success. While numerous and varied transformational strategies are proposed as improvement opportunities, attention must be focused on the use of valid and tested processes and tools. The processes and tools should support options for systems improvement and sustainability, avenues to integrate changes in organizational culture, or how one process or tool interfaces with the other concurrent and subsequent transformational project and program efforts (Vest & Gamm, 2009).

Using the best available evidence and quality improvement methods adds dimension and **value** to managing projects. Improving outcomes with a focus on the process and context of the organization and its systems are the ultimate goals of projects and program development. Identifying change champions, opinion leaders, and key stakeholders provides the momentum for moving plans along. Knowing how to challenge the process and influence the outcome are also important to the dissemination, diffusion, and sustainability of the effort. Porter-O'Grady and Malloch (2009) stated that leaders must facilitate change, manage risk, eliminate irrelevance, create innovative teams, and provide visionary leadership to effectively move organizations forward regardless of the project initiative.

Any newly conceptualized or redesigned healthcare project requires the developer to first consider the organizational culture and its readiness for change in relation to the project. Additionally, Kaplin (2009) advocated the need to consider the nature of communication within a system or organization, communicate problems, identify needs related to communication problems, and develop strategies for enhancing communication between and among staff and within the entire system. A series of steps can assist staff when planning for redesign of a system and include the following:

- Complete a readiness assessment.
- Establish the perspectives for redesign.

- Create a standardized format for the redesign process.
- Gather internal and external data.
- Choose tools that will support redesign plans (Bolman & Deal, 2003; Bossidy & Charan, 2004; Kotter, 1996; Weick, 2001).

Examples of clinical redesign efforts may include the following:

- Integration of mental health in primary care.
- Implementation of an open access system for more clinic appointments.
- Primary care redesign.
- Development of a structured outreach program that enhances care coordination and meets the needs of vulnerable populations.

Practice changes require organizational culture changes. A lasting change rarely happens without consideration of the organization's culture and structure. Pivotal to the project's successful start and sustainability is the impact it will have within a multilayered health system. Organizational culture reviews and assessment tools are important to this end.

Project planning would be incomplete without considering the *whats* of the project. Thinking (or rethinking) what one needs (or desires) to do provides additional insights to the process. Merrifield (2009) poses the following questions for this rethinking process:

1. Does it directly correlate with any of your organization's key business goals? For example, does it resolve a customer's question or problem?
2. Does it have a strong connection to the organization's brand or corporate identity?
3. Is an effort to increase the performance of the *what* likely to cause it to become high(er) value?

If there are high value and low performers involved in what the project planner believes needs to be changed, serious attention must be paid to the process and anticipated outcomes. If the project change is of high value with high performers, monitoring progress may be all that is needed to make changes. Low value and low performance changes may direct the project leader to consider automation, outsourcing, or even a decision to abandon the change altogether. This may also be true of low value and high performers as they may be considered a major waste of resources. These points are critical to the sustainability of any planned change.

A market feasibility study is an adjunct to questions posed by Merrifield (The Strategic Performance Group, 2009). Market feasibility studies are composed of two sections—when to conduct a study and the study process components. When conducting a market feasibility study there are three considerations. These include:

1. Launching a new project or product.
2. Offering a new service with a program or system.
3. Considering opening a new program or facility.

The feasibility study process focuses on the following four areas:

1. Profile of the desired demographics of the project or program target market.
2. Assessment of competitors to determine their strengths and weaknesses.
3. Identification of the market opportunities.
4. Survey of prospective customer base potential for use of new or expanded services that will be offered.

Other questions to consider involve how the organization/system is currently performing. The project director asks the following questions:

- How is it currently performing?
- Do we know and understand what causes performance today?
- Do we know and understand what it would take to improve performance? (Merrifield, 2009).

As the organization's culture is examined, levels within the system must be considered. Nelson, Batalden, and Godfrey (2007) pointedly captured this notion and espoused that the project developer must consider three principal levels in a typical integrated delivery system. The three levels include the macrosystem, the mesosystem, and the microsystem. The macrosystem is the whole of the organization led by senior leadership, whereas the mesosystem constitutes the major divisions of the organization. The microsystem is the small units where individuals provide services (Nelson, Batalden, & Godfrey, 2007). Depending on the depth of the project, focusing on a particular level may be the emphasis of one's work. For example, a clinical nurse leader focuses on projects at the clinical microsystem. The projects may be as varied as reducing length of stay on a surgical trauma unit, reducing costs of care, or decreasing readmission rates. The executive nurse administrator and doctor of nursing practice student or graduate may focus on projects at the mesosystem or macrosystem. At the mesosytem, projects such as developing department-wide programs for mother and baby care to improve continuity of care and patient satisfaction are examples. Developing a clinical ladder for a hospital-wide nursing department is an example of a project at the macrosystem level.

Leadership is also cornerstone to successful projects and their management. Tushman and O'Reilly (1996) identified themes from high-performing leaders that include:

- Seeing the problem or opportunity.
- Willingness to change the present situation.
- Implementing the **innovation** for improved performance.
- Using design and reengineering methods to improve patient flow and work flow, while reducing inefficiencies and eliminating defects.

The real test of leadership, then, is to be able to compete successfully by both increasing the alignment or fit among strategy, structure, culture, and process, while simultaneously preparing for the inevitable revolutions through disconcerting environmental changes. This requires organizational and management skills to compete in a mature market where efficiency, cost, and incremental innovation are key, and to develop new products and services where radical innovation, speed, and flexibility are critical.

Project Planning and Program Management Overview

Completing any project—from the intuitive idea to the development of a business plan and its implementation—is rarely a linear process. It requires multiple skill sets, adaptability and flexibility, and the ability to simultaneously manage multiple other projects and programs. Complexity science and microsystems literature offer a perspective that focuses on interrelationships, interdependencies, and dynamic systems. Complexity science provides the language, metaphors, conceptual frameworks, models, and theories that help make the idiosyncrasies nonidiosyncratic and the illogical logical (Lindberg, Nash, & Lindberg, 2008). For some leaders who are studying complexity, the science is counterintuitive because of the stark contrast with what they had been taught about how organizations operate. Project planning takes this into account as strategies are brainstormed and determined to be value added.

Complexity science describes how systems actually behave, rather than how they should behave. Complexity science challenges one to examine the unpredictable, disorderly, and unstable aspects of organizations. Complexity complements our traditional understanding of organizations to provide us with a complete picture. Without this complete picture, project management falls short of providing the best and soundest ways to innovate for improvement (Lindberg, Nash, & Lindberg, 2008).

When planning projects within complex adaptive systems, greater insights can be gained into the project's context and value to a program or organization. Healthcare organizations are complex adaptive systems. What is a complex adaptive system? The three words in the name are each significant in the definition. *Complex* implies diversity—a great number of connections between wide varieties of elements. *Adaptive* suggests the capacity to alter or change—the ability to learn from experience. A *system* is a set of connected or interdependent things. The things in a complex adaptive system are independent agents. An agent may be a person, a molecule, a species, or an organization, or one of many others (Plsek, 2003).

Leadership is a central element of project management and program development. Knowing how to engage and inspire others to sustain improvement changes in systems defines the leadership role. Leadership considers the strategy, structure, culture, and processes while simultaneously preparing for the inevitable revolutions required by discontinuous environmental change. Organizational and management skills are increasingly important in order to compete in today's market. According to Tushman and O'Reilly (1996), project managers must be both organized and able to manage multiple things simultaneously while focusing on an identified project. That is, they must be ambidextrous. This textbook will address project management and development from strategy, structure, culture, and processes that are integral to a system and success.

Advancing leadership in project planning is critical to a productive team and sustaining positive outcomes. Porter-O'Grady and Malloch (2009) describe leadership and levels of emergence in complex systems. They describe major competencies related to network leadership in innovative organizations. Such competencies include an understanding of the key drivers of change within health care, the ability to connect to the core work of the healthcare enterprise, scanning skills related to the confluence of forces in the external environment and highly leveraged translational skills in adaptive external–internal integration challenges as they reconceptualize the character and content of health service (p. 13). Group work also constitutes a level of emergence in complex systems. Innovative process techniques include the following: nominal process, action lists, brainstorming, forced choice, jigsaw learning, Delphi technique, strategy maps, social judgment analysis, cognitive maps, role defined, and sticky note boards.

> A common characteristic of the leader of innovation is the ability and high-level skill in the act of synchronicity. Real-time collaborative and synchronous coordination of the various operating characteristics, strategy, structure, processes, and human dynamics is a strong indicator of effectiveness in complex adaptive systems. (Porter-O'Grady & Malloch, 2009, p. 27).

Thinking inside the box is also a strategy and works nicely with thinking outside the box. Becoming competent in both makes positive deviance more apparent. Porter-O'Grady and Malloch (2010) identify inside-the-box behaviors for positive deviants, which include recognizing that leaders cannot possibly have all the answers or always ask the best questions, nurture and encourage others to ask questions, recognize the value of the team, look at others with a different lens, and be fully engaged (p. 47). Facilitating the creative project requires guidelines to the innovative process. Points to consider are: being flexible, being open, embracing failures, being creative, abandoning ego, exploring differences, being resilient, enjoying oneself, exploring technology, and coaching (p. 56).

Another viewpoint of project management may be considered from three perspectives:

1. Technical
2. Context
3. Value-added

The technical perspective includes the didactics of project planning, development, and management. This outlook will consider the techniques useful in determining the need for the project (making the compelling case; needs assessment), steps in developing, planning, and evaluating the outcomes. Additionally, deciding on the best metrics from a qualitative and quantitative point of view is also included. Determining sound evidence to support a project is outlined as an important component for project implementation. A project developer must give consideration to seeking institutional review board approval during the needs assessment process. Institutional review board approval allows data collected to be disseminated beyond the scope of the assessment project in the organization and is advantageous when communicating findings and successes to external audiences and forums.

Considering the context and processes of project management focuses on the infrastructure, organizational culture, stakeholders, and evidence-based framework for improvement changes. Change theory, innovation, and implementation science are explored in context to the project undertaken.

Value-added refers to finding the meaning in the overall project. It is the determination of what matters. It is the *so what?* of the project idea. Without knowing the importance of doing the project and what value the work will add, one may miss the larger context of the plan. This aspect of project planning is critical to defining real outcomes based on the value the project adds to the overall system. Morris (2009) stated the key to understanding the business value of a project or program is looking past standard metrics. Morris stated this can be accomplished by asking and answering these 10 questions:

1. What is the overall value of the project for the entire organization?
2. What is the overall value for a department?
3. What is the overall value for customers and stakeholders?
4. What is the overall cost of the project, possible alternatives to reducing cost, the return on investment, and the payback period of the initial project investment?
5. What is the priority or rank of the proposed project in relation to others under consideration in a specific department or division?
6. What is the overall rank of the project in relation to all projects in the system or organization?
7. What risks are associated with the project?
8. Does the organization have the capacity to begin and complete the project?
9. What is the scoring methodology used to select the project over others?
10. What processes are in place to override other proposed projects if the one being proposed is not ranked high or approved?

The project idea may be a raw idea that could become an elegant solution to a challenging problem or an authentic something better, thus improving the overall situation. Creating new solutions may not be enough to solve problems. Making things better can be achieved by making distinctions, seeing versus looking and elegance. Understanding the cause(s) provides important means to identify outcomes and **evaluation** tools. It is knowing the what, how, and why that leads to better problem solving and decision making (Sindell, 2009). Sindell offered ways to think creatively, focusing on innovation.

> Creative thought is about looking at what everyone is looking at, or has looked at for years, and seeing something new. Sometimes that new thing is just the possibility of something new, and sometimes what we see is right in there, already in existence, but has never been noticed before. (Sindell, 2009, p. 15)

Sindell also considered complexity, simplicity, and elegance.

> When we have refined our thinking to the point that our hard work has become invisible, then we will have achieved elegance. Elegance is not only good ideas well thought through, but also, good ideas cleaned up and well dressed. Elegant thinking is much more likely to be invited in. (Sindell, 2009, p. 18)

This book will provide opportunities for the reader to work through refinement of ideas by ongoing testing against the writer's original intent, need, and vision by making careful note of shortfalls and further refining the work. Sindell (2009) stated, "the better our observational skills, the better our interview skills, the faster we can refine our ideas as we get closer to our original intent" (p. 53). The more one is steeped in his practice, organizational culture, and leadership and has the skills to uncover, discover, and make distinction as to the originality of the work, the greater likelihood of success and sustainability. Sindell additionally offered the genius machine model. These 11 steps (pp. 131–133) may be useful in turning raw ideas into elegant solutions. These include:

1. Distinctions: What do I see?
2. Identity: Who am I? Why are these ideas important to me, and why am I driven to share them with the world?
3. Implications: Where do my ideas lead?
4. Testing: Have I questioned everything about my assumptions?
5. Precedent: Who else has seen something like this?
6. Need: Who needs this knowledge? This question forces us out of focusing solely on our own area and may lead us to find the universals in our thinking.

7. Foundation: Are there underlying principles? What are the underlying values expressed here? What are the applicable rules or structures that we obtain here?
8. Completion: Is everything here?
9. Connecting: Whom am I addressing? Do I understand my audience's frame of reference?
10. Impact: Where do I want to go? Will this project take on a life of its own?
11. Advocacy: Am I supporting the adoption of my ideas? My thinking stands for me. Now I must stand for what I have created.

Thinking through this frame of reference and asking such questions leads to a clearer way of imagining ideas and how to make them real.

Understanding the various conceptual and theoretical perspectives will be integrated into the foundations of project planning and **program management** and will be discussed in Chapter 2. Void of guiding principles, explaining and justifying a need for a project or program is difficult. The purpose of the project can become obtuse and be subject to rigorous debate, and the organization may question its funding. In effect, as the project is planned, transparency and linkage of the purpose to a mission that enhances value and engenders participation by others cannot be overstated.

Chapter 3 ("Requisite Competencies and Skills for Effective Project Planning and Program Management") will detail the requisite competencies and skills for effective project planning and program management. Investment in skill set development by organizations can be realized as projects' desired outcomes occur and as quality milestones are achieved. To this end, a control process must be part of the project's life cycle so variances can be managed and project aims are attained. Effective governance can often assist in the overall direction of a project, further validating the need for new skill sets by others.

Chapter 4 ("Team Power and Synergy: Project Planning and Program Management Essentials") captures the importance of teams, team synergy, and strategies that support value-added team techniques.

Chapter 5 ("Planning a Project for Implementation") discusses the steps in planning a sustainable project and the life cycle of a project plan. Additionally, the chapter discusses how a system's need is identified from the microsystem, mesosystem, and macrosystem perspectives. Project risks and how to manage them are addressed, as are stakeholders' roles in supporting a project or program.

Without addressing risks and potential vulnerabilities, projects may not be funded, stated, or survive in a constantly changing and turbulent environment. Chapter 6 ("The Needs Assessment: Foundations for Clinical Application") expands on information discussed in Chapter 4 about the needs assessment and the SWOT analysis. The chapter further provides an overview of steps in completing a clinical needs assessment and techniques that support the process both for organizations and communities. Considerations about submitting an institutional review board application and a sample are provided.

Chapter 7 ("Implementing a Project") discusses the steps to take when implementing a project, the value of collaboration, and actions of the project manager. The importance of communication is offered as an essential component for project success. A systems change model is outlined to assist in sustaining projects and support programs.

Chapter 8 ("The Role of Information Technology and the Enterprise in Project Planning and Implementation") introduces how information technology and the enterprise drive decisions and ultimate success of a project. Examples of clinical projects are the processes associated with development and implementation and are detailed in this chapter.

Chapter 9 ("Developing Metrics That Support Projects and Programs") identifies methods that support projects and programs, tools for assessing organizational culture and the relationship to a project or program, and how to ascribe meaning to data. Step-by-step approaches are offered. Differentiating various stages and levels of change and innovation are underscored, including diffusion, dissemination, implementation, and sustainability. Knowing what works and how it works is required for project and program success.

Measuring the value of projects within organizations is captured in Chapter 10. The value of a project requires one to use information that is available and that captures the stakeholders' interest. Thus, efficiencies and inefficiencies are measured in terms of value assigned to a project, and metrics can be aligned for ongoing valuation.

Chapter 11 ("Evaluating Project Outcomes") discusses data analysis techniques in project management and the importance of outcomes in forecasting future organizational performance.

Chapter 12 ("Disseminating Results as a Mechanism for Sustaining Innovation") includes a discussion of mechanisms that communicate project outcomes that are pivotal to sustainability of projects or making them stick. Additionally, sustainability is enhanced by professionally presenting the project to groups and stakeholders as detailed in this chapter.

Chapters 13 and 14 (both titled "Voices from the Field," but with different subtitles) provide examples of clinical practice projects, faculty, assignment examples, faculty dialogue, and student projects from nurse executive, clinical nurse leader, and doctor of nursing practice students.

But what differentiates project planning and program management, and why must projects complement existing or planned programs? Projects are temporary and have unique products or services. They should add value to the organization. As one plans a project, four phases occur: initiation, planning, implementation, and closeout (ESI, 2008). Attention to what resources are needed and which must be mobilized to activate a project is essential to valued outcomes and impact. Whether it is a student planning a capstone project or a skilled administrator, projects that will have sustainable impact on areas beyond the initial months should be developed. This is where the skilled and transformational leader incorporates innovation into project planning. The innovation further supports the overall mission of an organization, while effectively utilizing multiple avenues to attain a stated goal and objectives. Avenues to monitor successes and adjust as needed are pivotal as programs are managed. An example of how a student project can lead to sustainable outcomes is when an administrator who is managing a care delivery division adopts the student's project, as illustrated in **Box 1-1**.

Box 1-1   Sustaining Student Projects in a Nursing Division

Based on a gap analysis, a graduate student and the unit director identify missed opportunities where additional outpatient appointments could be added each clinic day. The student develops a capstone project whereby add-on appointments are available for walk-in patients each morning and afternoon based on an analysis of provider downtime and clinic operation hours. The project is implemented with much success. The unit director continues to monitor productivity following the student's graduation and through some additional modifications, opens additional slots resulting in clinic efficiency and increased profits.

Using Concept Analysis as a Tool When Developing Sustainable Projects

An initial step in formulating a project is considering the **organizational readiness** for change, its adaptability, and the meaningfulness of the project to the overall mission of a system. Readying the environment includes creating a sense of urgency. Influence and relationship-based persuasion can be powerful tools in fostering an environment that embraces innovation. Branding strategies provide the how-to of what can and must be done when creating coalitions that support a project and its sustainability.

As the project begins, a systematic process called a concept analysis can prove useful (Walker & Avant, 1995). The process includes identification of the antecedents, consequences, and outcomes. Antecedents are the events or incidents that occur prior to a project being planned or implemented. Consequences follow and are defined as the events or incidents that occur as a result of the project. Outcomes are the sustainable results that continuously support the efficacy of a program managed by a designated staff or leader within an organization. **Table 1-1** provides an example of process as it relates to project planning and program management.

Table 1-1   Project Planning and Program Management Antecedents, Consequences, and Outcomes for Elective Surgery Cancellations

Antecedents	Consequences	Outcomes
Balanced score card revealed elective surgery cancellations exceeding targets by 20%.	Process action team organized and project development targeted at reducing elective surgery cancellations and efficiency.	Continuous efficacy and efficiency.
Loss of revenue for 2 cycles.		Staff and patient satisfaction increased and maintained.
Decreased patient satisfaction.		
Decreased staff satisfaction.	Patient surgical workups complete.	Intra- and interdisciplinary communication enhanced.
Surgery schedule unpredictable with heavy and light days.	Equipment/supplies available.	
Supply department efficiency reduced and costs spiraling.	Surgery schedule distributed equitably throughout the week with options for emergency add-on cases.	Elective surgery cancellations reduced from 55% to 14%.
Surgery equipment not readily available.		

Beyond the concept, analysis process is asking, what is the value of the project to the overall programs within a system, and what is its sustainability power? Value can be assigned to a project and measured as it is sustained over time. But how does one ensure the project will be of value and can be sustained? Visible involvement of senior management is essential to sustaining projects and their overall contribution to programs and healthcare environments (McGrath et al., 2008). Of equal importance is engaging other leaders and staff. Gaining trust of staff and including them early in the project development is important. Establishing targets and attainable time frames will assist in managing the project and maintaining improvements. Projects are likely to be sustained if they evidence documented outcomes (Akerlund, 2000). Backer (2000) stated projects are more easily managed and sustained when they include user-friendly communication that is understood, when they allow for easy access, and when they have external (community/stakeholder) involvement.

The Relationship Among Innovation, Project, and Program Management

Healthcare executives are hardwired to manage multiple priorities and projects. Therefore, the project developer and implementer must be similarly hardwired. As projects are developed and implemented, a myriad of accommodation must also occur. The project designer and manager must accommodate to the needs of an evolving or static system and various cultural dynamics, and executives must adapt to the change inherent in a new or redesigned project, the interrelatedness, and interwoven threads. The mission, vision, and values of an organization also cannot be dismissed and should be easily recognized in the project. This allows for continuity and can be leveraged to involve other disciplines to participate and assist in sustaining the identified project.

Everett Rogers (1995) has been instrumental in the work of innovation. He identified the following 10 factors that influence the progression of innovation:

1. Relative advantage: What value does the innovation bring to the system?
2. Tryability: Can the innovation be tried out or trialed?
3. Observability: Is the innovation seen by others?
4. Communication channels: What specific channels do opinion leaders and early adopters use to transmit their experience, outcomes, and opinions in their local social networks and more distant connections?

5. Homophilous groups: What are key characteristics of the target group? Are they homogeneous?
6. Pace of innovation/reinvention: Is it easy to adapt to the innovation?
7. Norms, roles, social networks: Are there homogeneous connections? Distant connections?
8. Opinion leaders: Who are your most influential and respected individuals?
9. Compatibility: How aligned is the innovation with the user's current knowledge, skills, attitudes, and beliefs?
10. Infrastructure support: What is the existing structure, and is it strong to support the innovation?

Using the questions to guide project ideas and eventual project development can be useful in considering value-added innovations.

As discussed in Chapter 12, it is important to identify tools useful for making it stick. It is not uncommon for great innovative projects to be developed and successful while a leader remains in a current position or organization. However, when the leader leaves the environment, all too often, the innovation slowly disintegrates. Christensen and Raynor (2003) stated the key to sustaining an innovation is to target demanding high-end users with sustained and better outcomes. Thus, it is the *who* the innovator targets that becomes the key to sustainability. Sindell (2009) offered ways to think creatively, focusing on innovation. Sometimes thinking creatively allows one to see something new that was already in existence and never noticed before, further sustaining an innovative idea or project.

Summary

- Planning and implementing projects require a rigorous series of actions.
- Practice changes require organizational culture change.
- Project developers and implementers must consider three levels in a delivery system: macrosystem, mesosystem, and microsystem.
- Leadership is a cornerstone to successful projects and sustainability.
- Managing projects requires technical expertise, context of the how-to, and knowledge of the value or meaning in the overall project.
- Implementing a project requires consideration of organizational readiness.
- Concept analysis can be a useful tool in developing a sustainable project.
- Sustaining a project requires targeting the high-end user with sustained and better outcomes.

Suggested Readings

Godin, S. (2008). *Tribes: We need you to lead us.* New York: Penguin Group.

Kotter, J. (2008). *A sense of urgency.* Boston: Harvard Business School Publishing.

Shell, G. R., & Moussa, M. (2007). *The art of woo: Using strategic persuasion to sell your ideas.* New York: Penguin Group.

Reflection Questions

1. What elements and/or variables are attributed to sustainable projects and their impact on a healthcare system's sustained success and efficacy?
2. Sustainability can be attributed to multiple factors. What are general factors that can be attributed to project sustainability within organizations?
3. What makes a project elegant? How can these elements be integrated into your project plan?
4. What factors contribute to diffusing innovation? How can these factors add value to project ideas?

References

Akerlund, K. M. (2000). Prevention program sustainability: The state's perspective. *Journal of Community Psychology, 28*(3), 353–362.

Backer, T. E. (2000). The failure of success: Challenges of disseminating effective substance abuse programs. *Journal of Community Psychology, 28*(3), 363–373.

Christensen, C., & Raynor, M. (2003). *The innovator's solution.* Boston: Harvard Business School Press.

ESI. (2008). *Project management.* Arlington, VA: ESI International.

Kaplin, D. W. (2009). *Organizational communication: A needs assessment.* (ERIC Document Reproduction Service No. ED175071). Retrieved from http://www.eric.ed.gov:80/ERICWebPortal/custom/portlets/recordDetails/detailmini.jsp?_nfpb=true&_&ERICExtSearch_SearchValue_0=ED175071&ERICExtSearch_SearchType_0=no&accno=ED175071

Lindberg, C., Nash, S., & Lindberg, C. (2008). *On the edge: Nursing in the age of complexity.* Bordentown, NJ: Plexus Press.

McGrath, K. M., Bennett, D. M., Ben-Tovim, K. I., Boyages, S. C., Lyons, N. J., & O'Connell, T. J. (2008). Implementing and sustaining transformational change in health care: Lessons learnt about clinical process redesign. *The Medical Journal of Australia, 188*(6), 32–35.

Merrifield, R. (2009). *Re-think.* Upper Saddle River, NJ: Pearson.

Morris, R. A. (2009). *Project management that works!* [Web blog post]. Retrieved from http://www.pmthatworks.com/2009/12/determining-business-value-for-projects.html

Nelson, E., Batalden, P., & Godfrey, M. (2007). *Quality by design.* San Francisco: Jossey-Bass.

Plsek, P. (2003). *Complexity and the adoption of innovation in health care.* Paper presented at Accelerating Quality Improvements in Health Care: Strategies to Accelerate the Diffusion of Evidence-based Innovations, Washington, DC.

Porter-O'Grady, T., & Malloch, K. (2009). Leaders of innovation: Transforming postindustrial healthcare. *Journal of Nursing Administration, 39*(6), 245–248.

Porter-O'Grady, T., & Malloch, K. (2010). *Innovation leadership: Creating the leadership of health care.* Sudbury, MA: Jones and Bartlett.

Rogers, E. (1995). *Diffusion of innovation.* New York: Free Press.

Sindell, G. (2009). *The genius machine.* Novata, CA: New World Library.

Strategic Performance Group, LLC. (2009). Make sure your idea is sound: Investigate before investing. *Market Feasibility Studies.* Retrieved from http://www.spg-consulting.com/consulting-services/market-feasibility-studies?gclid=CPq

Tushman, M., & O'Reilly, C. (1996). The ambidextrous organization: managing evolutionary and revolutionary change. *California Management Review, 38*(4), 8–30.

Vest, J. R., & Gamm, L. D. (2009). A critical review of the research literature on Six Sigma, Lean and StuderGroup's Hardwiring Excellence in the United States: the need to demonstrate and communicate the effectiveness of transformation strategies in healthcare. *Implementation Science, 4*(35), 1–9.

Walker, L., & Avant, K. (Eds.). (1995). Concept analysis. In *Strategies for theory construction in nursing* (3rd ed., pp. 37–54). Norwalk, CT: Appleton & Lange.

TWO

Foundations of Project Planning and Program Management

■ Sandra E. Walters

■ **Learning Objectives**

1. Discuss conceptual and theoretical underpinnings of project planning and program management.
2. Identify ways to incorporate concepts and theory into project planning and program management.
3. Identify key elements that drive the development of a project and future management of programs.

"No institution can possibly survive if it needs geniuses or supermen to manage it. It must be organized in such a way as to be able to get along under a leadership composed of average human beings."

—Peter F. Drucker

Key Terms

Complexity

Human factors engineering

Innovations

Program management

Project planning

Quality improvement

Transparency

Value

Roles

Advocate

Communicator

Decision maker

Integrator

Leader

Risk anticipator

Professional Values

Altruism

Evidence-based practice

Integrity

Patient-centric care

Quality

Social justice

Core Competencies

Appreciative inquiry

Assessment

Coordination

Critical thinking

Design

Emotional intelligence

Health promotion

Interpersonal influence

Leadership

Management

Resource management

Risk reduction

Systems thinking

Introduction

A prerequisite for **project planning** and **program management** is a reasonable belief that changes will result from interventions undertaken, and that the changes will occur in a somewhat predictable manner. While the underlying assumptions may not be recognized as constituting a conceptual or theoretical framework, the expectation of cause and effect is present and forms the basis for both project planning and program management. The theoretical foundation for nursing is essential to the planning process as one attempts to explain nursing practice.

Conceptual Models and Theoretical Frameworks

Multiple attempts have been made to define the phenomena of interest to the discipline of nursing. These metaparadigms are the most abstract intellectual and social missions of the discipline and have been developed to explain what the boundaries of nursing are, what nursing's core concepts are, and how these are interrelated (Fawcett, 2004). The core concepts identified by the National League for Nursing and later refined by Fawcett as being central to nursing are human beings, environment, health, and nursing. These concepts are defined and linked by relational propositions such that human beings are the participants in nursing; the environment is composed of the individuals who surround the participants as well as conditions associated with health; health is a process of living and dying; and nursing includes all actions taken by nurses on the patient's behalf (Fawcett). Because the metaparadigm is an abstract and global view of what the concerns of the discipline are, it does not provide the directions needed for research and practice. The foundation for research and practice is, instead, found in the theories and conceptual models of nursing (Alligood & Marriner-Tobey, 2006).

Like metaparadigms, conceptual models are composed of concepts and the statements that link them. Walker and Avant (2005, p. 26) defined concepts as "expressions used to provide mental images of a phenomenon, an idea, or a construct about a thing or an action." Fawcett (2004) referred to the statements of the relation between concepts as propositions. These concepts and the propositions that link them can provide a framework for general and abstract ideas and thus a way to think about and understand reality. When a conceptual model is used for development of relatively concrete and specific concepts linked by relatively concrete relations, theory is developed (Fawcett). Van Sell and Kalofissidus (2001) characterized nursing theories as essential to the socialization of nurses into the profession. These nursing theories provide language, identify important concepts, define relationships, facilitate communication, and predict the outcomes of nursing practice. In this manner, models are derived from theories and are used to demonstrate how a theory can be applied to practice.

A concept analysis of a theoretical framework or model provides an understanding of the attributes of concepts, presents operational definitions with a clear theoretical basis, and can facilitate instrument development for project planning and program management (Rodgers & Knafl, 2000; Walker & Avant, 2005). The philosophic foundations for the analysis of concepts have been the subject of rigorous debate and form the basis for discussions on how knowledge is developed (Chinn & Kramer, 1999; Creasia & Parker, 2007; Malloch & Porter-O'Grady, 2006; Rodgers & Knafl, 2000). Since a project involves development of a plan of action for a specific purpose, the purpose is often a central concept. In other words, the first step in project planning is the selection of a phenomenon of interest. The selection is often based on factors such as the individual interests, values, resources, available time, and the view of nursing of the individual planner (Chinn & Kramer, 1999). Once a concept is identified, an examination of the concept proceeds with a literature search related to the concept selected.

From a literature search, research related to the concept may lead to theoretical frameworks and models that have been used to define the concept. One need only examine any dictionary to realize that words frequently have multiple meanings and that their meaning is often dependent on the context in which a word is used. Defining the concept using a selected theory helps to keep consistency between the theoretical framework and the language while providing a basis for linking relationship statements to expected outcomes (Houser, 2008; Morse, 2000). In this manner, the use of theory to guide practice fulfills the requirement that project planning and program management be based on a sound theoretical framework and provides a contextual frame of reference for the concept in question. By reflecting on nursing theories, nurses can identify what they believe are the essential elements of the nursing process and ensure consistency between their concept and the propositions of their selected theory. Theories such as Newman's theory of expanding consciousness, Peplau's theory of interpersonal relations, and Parse's theory of human beçoming are among the many that can be found in the literature (Fawcett, 2004; Creasia & Parker, 2007). Houser (2007) outlined three steps for use in evaluating whether a theoretical framework has been used in a study in a manner consistent with the original theory (**Table 2-1**). The steps can also be used when critiquing a project.

From the initial examination of the theoretical framework and concepts of a project, refinement of ideas occurs. The successful application of the framework in prior studies is noted together with any necessary refinements required for application to the project at hand. The framework will help to identify measures for use in validating the outcomes of the project or program being undertaken.

Table 2-1   Steps for Critiquing a Study Theory and Projects

Step 1—Extract all concepts and their definitions from the framework and find them in the research study; examine them for consistency and whether each has a reference from the literature.

Step 2—Determine the relationships between concepts, how they are analyzed and validated; compare these to the theorist's definitions and references.

Step 3—Determine if the researcher's claims are supported by the framework and whether the framework explains the phenomena and relationships presented.

Source: Houser, 2007, p. 173.

Key Drivers of Project Planning and Program Management

For nurses to address the demands of technology and the changing needs of patients in the complex healthcare system, they must be prepared to coordinate and integrate care provided by nursing and others (Mitchell, 2008). This can be achieved through project planning and program management, which provide a mechanism to address a task or problem within a specified time frame and using allocated resources. In effect, the drivers for well-executed project planning and program management are the need for nurses' participation in implementing **innovations**, improving quality, providing **transparency**, enhancing **value**, and dealing with **complexity** in health care. An examination of these key drivers is useful in understanding the context in which planning will occur.

Innovation can be defined as the introduction of a new idea, method, or product as a deliberate application of knowledge, imagination, and initiative such that risk taking and a different value result (Vereck & Beck, 2009). Evaluation of the implementation of new technology for diagnosing and treating illness is essential as project outcomes are realized. There are six critical elements for safety in health services identified by the Institute of Medicine (IOM) that can be used to evaluate innovations. These are the qualities of patient safety, effectiveness, timeliness, patient-centric efficiency, and equity (Steinwachs & Hughes, 2008). One strategy for achieving the safety goals has been the application of **human factors engineering** in the healthcare arena. This scientific discipline examines human characteristics and how humans interact with the world around them and apply the principles, data, and methods to optimize system performance (Powell-Cope, Nelson, & Patterson, 2008).

Quality improvement is another driver of project planning and program management that can be evaluated on the basis of the IOM safety goals. Quality improvement can be defined as systematic, data-guided activity that produces immediate improvement in healthcare delivery in specified settings as a means of reducing a quality gap (Hughes, 2008). Multiple strategies for improving quality have been identified, including total quality management, zero defects, six sigma, and Baldrige quality improvement. While the choice of strategies depends on the nature of the project, the general premise is that a process that needs improvement is identified, key performance measures are determined, a new process is developed based on an in-depth analysis, the refined process is implemented, and performance is reassessed to determine if improvement has occurred (Hughes). While quality improvement initiatives often result in organization-specific data, the strategies for the projects may be employed as a means to achieve the safety goals of the IOM.

Transparency as a driver for project planning and program management refers to the availability of information from insurers, providers, hospitals, and other healthcare organizations including care pricing, quality, resource utilization, outcomes, and performance indicators to the decision makers or consumers of health care (Azar, Miller, Kendall, & Francis, 2007). The assumption is that if information were made available, competition would lead to lower prices and improved quality. In similar manner, healthcare value as an economic driver refers to the ability of the healthcare system to compete in terms of pricing for goods and services. Additionally, healthcare value has a social, political, and cultural aspect that refers to factors in a healthcare system such as the education level of the nursing staff, the degree to which practitioners have specialty certifications, and even the level of employee satisfaction (Malloch & Porter-O'Grady, 2006). In effect, factors that influence the ability of institutions to recruit and retain the most skilled and educated healthcare professionals can provide an impetus for change and the need for project planning and program management.

The inherent complexity of the healthcare system has been portrayed as leading to system failures, producing a high-risk environment, and causing deficiencies in the ability to solve problems (Scott, 2006). Characteristics of complex systems that lead to breakdowns include system parts that produce unplanned interactions, tight coupling of interactions whereby precision must be present, conflicting goals at many levels of the organization, fluid participation by uninformed or uninterested actors, and rapid changes that are not in the control of the system (Scott, 2006). When planning projects and managing programs, complexity science provides a mechanism for understanding the complex healthcare system and explains how results are not linear as with mechanistic systems where small changes produce minimal results.

Complexity science in nursing was derived in the 1990s from chaos and is based on the philosophical belief that the future is not predictable and the whole is not simply a sum of parts. The model places value on the adaptability of living systems, intuitive understanding, unpredictability of life, self-organizing agencies, and outcomes that are nonlinear patterns of relationships (Burns, 2001). Human beings, the environment, health, and nursing are seen as a dynamic, living, and complex adaptive system where diversity and variability help to ensure adaptability and development. As energy or other inputs impact the open complex adaptive systems, disequilibrium is sustained as life with a complex pattern of change, growth, and learning (Zimmerman, Lindberg, & Plsek, 1998). Program managers will be most effective when they establish relationships among people, ensure diversity in work groups, allow action to emerge from the front lines, and begin with small things that work and then link successful aspects to form more complex systems (Burns, 2001). Essentially, spending less time on tight control and more time on relationships supports greater sustainability, a key consideration when planning projects and managing programs.

Summary

- Planning and implementing projects require a solid theoretical framework.
- The foundation for research and practice is theories and conceptual models.
- Identification of measures for evaluation of concepts must be developed from the basis of a theoretical framework or conceptual model.
- Drivers of project planning and program management in health care arise from innovations, quality improvement, transparency, value, and complexity.
- Healthcare systems are living entities with the ability to adapt.

Suggested Readings

Alligood, M. R., & Marriner-Tomey, A. (2006). *Nursing theory: Utilization & application* (3rd ed.). St. Louis, MO: Mosby.

Hardin, S., & Kaplow, R. (2005). *Synergy for clinical excellence: The AACN synergy model for patient care*. Sudbury, MA: Jones and Bartlett.

Jarrín, O. F. (2007). An integral philosophy and definition of nursing. *AQAL: Journal of Integral Theory and Practice, 2*(4), 79–101.

Marriner-Tomey, A., & Alligood, M. R. (2006). *Nursing theorists and their work* (6th ed.). St. Louis, MO: Mosby.

Meleis, A. I. (2007). *Theoretical nursing: Development and progress* (4th ed.). Philadelphia: Lippincott.

Nightingale, F. (1969). *Notes on nursing* (Original publication in 1859). Mineola, NY: Dover Publications.

Parker, M. (2006). *Nursing theorists and their application in practice* (2nd ed.). Philadelphia: F. A. Davis.

Peterson, S. J., & Bredow, T. S. (2004). *Middle range theories: Application to nursing theory*. Philadelphia: Lippincott Williams & Wilkins.

Sieloff, C. L., & Frey, M. (2007). *Middle range theories from within Imogene King's interacting systems framework*. New York: Springer.

Reflection Questions

1. Identify two nursing theories and compare the way each views the concepts of humans, the environment, health, and nursing.
2. The need for project planning and program management can be driven by internal as well as external factors in healthcare systems. Identify factors that would drive changes for internal stakeholders.

Learning Activity

Select a research study from the literature and identify the theoretical framework used by the researcher. Include a list of concepts and their definitions as outlined in Table 2-1 to critique the study.

References

Alligood, M. R., & Marriner-Tomey, A. (2006). *Nursing theory: Utilization and application* (3rd ed.). St. Louis, MO: Mosby.

Azar, A. M., Miller, T. P., Kendall, D. B., & Francis, W. (2007). *Transparency in health care: What consumers need to know*. Retrieved from http://www.heritage.org/research/healthcare /hl986.cfm

Burns, J. P. (2001). Complexity science and leadership in healthcare. *Journal of Nursing Administration, 31*(10), 474–482.

Chinn, P., & Kramer, M. (1999). *Theory and nursing: Integrated knowledge development* (7th ed.). St. Louis, MO: Mosby.

Creasia, J. L., & Parker, B. J. (2007). *Conceptual foundations: The bridge to professional nursing practice* (4th ed.). St. Louis, MO: Mosby.

Fawcett, J. (2004). *Contemporary nursing knowledge: Analysis and evaluation of nursing models and theories* (2nd ed.). Philadelphia: F. A. Davis.

Houser, J. (2007). *Nursing research: Reading, using and creating evidence*. Sudbury, MA: Jones and Bartlett.

Hughes, R. G. (2008). Tools and strategies for quality improvement and patient safety. In R. G. Hughes (Ed.), *Patient safety and quality: An evidence-based handbook for nurses* (Vol. 1). Rockville, MD: Agency for Healthcare Research and Quality.

Malloch, K., & Porter-O'Grady, T. (Eds.). (2006). *Introduction to evidence-based practice in nursing and healthcare*. Sudbury, MA: Jones and Bartlett.

Mitchell, P. (2008). Defining patient safety and quality care. In R. G. Hughes (Ed.), *Patient safety and quality: An evidence-based handbook for nurses* (Vol. 1). Rockville, MD: Agency for Healthcare Research and Quality.

Morse, J. M. (2000). Exploring pragmatic utility: Concept analysis by critically appraising the literature. In B. L. Rodgers & K. A. Knafl (Eds.), *Concept development in nursing: Foundations, techniques and application* (2nd ed.). Philadelphia: Saunders.

Powell-Cope, G., Nelson, A. L., & Patterson, E. S. (2008). Patient care, technology and safety. In R. G. Hughes (Ed.), *Patient safety and quality: An evidence-based handbook for nurses* (Vol. 3). Rockville, MD: Agency for Healthcare Research and Quality.

Rodgers, B. L., & Knafl, K. A. (2000). *Concept development in nursing: Foundations, techniques and application* (2nd ed.). Philadelphia: Saunders.

Scott, K. A. (2006). Managing variance through an evidence-based framework for safe and reliable healthcare. In K. Malloch & T. Porter-O'Grady (Eds.), *Introduction to evidence-based practice in nursing and healthcare* (pp. 149–181). Sudbury, MA: Jones and Bartlett.

Steinwachs, D. M., & Hughes, R. G. (2008). Health services research: Scope and significance. In R. G. Hughes (Ed.), *Patient safety and quality: An evidence-based handbook for nurses* (Vol. 1). Rockville, MD: Agency for Healthcare Research and Quality.

Van Sell, S., & Kalofissudis, I. (2001). The evolving essence of the science of nursing: A complexity integration nursing theory. *ICUs and Nursing Web Journal, 8,* 3–25.

Vereck, B., & Beck, R. (2009). *Innovation.* Retrieved from http://www.businessdictionary.com/definition/innovation.html

Walker, L. O., & Avant, K. C. (2005). *Strategies for theory construction in nursing* (4th ed.). Upper Saddle River, NJ: Prentice Hall.

Zimmerman, B., Lindberg, C., & Plsek, P. (1998). A complexity science primer: What is complexity science and why should I learn about it? In *Edgeware: Lessons from complexity science for health care leaders.* Dallas, TX: VHA Inc.

THREE

Requisite Competencies and Skills for Effective Project Planning and Program Management

■ Mark Balch, Reji John, Kerrian Reynolds, and Cathy Rick

■ **Learning Objectives**

1. Identify core competencies and skill sets for managing projects and programs.
2. Link project plans to program management.
3. Compare program and project management.

> "Do not follow where the path may lead. Go instead where there is no path and leave a trail."
>
> —Ralph Waldo Emerson

Key Terms

Assessment	Leadership
Communication	Vision

Roles

Change champion	Leader
Communicator	Resource manager
Decision maker	

Professional Values

Integrity	Quality
Objectivity	

Core Competencies

Communication	Interpersonal influence
Coordination	Management
Critical thinking	Visionary leadership

Introduction

Project planning and program management are built upon the core elements of strategic planning at all levels of an organization. **Leadership** excellence demands skills and abilities for detailed project planning and results-oriented program management. Executive-level responsibilities focus on addressing today's challenges and opportunities while thinking ahead to develop approaches for efficient and effective nursing contributions. This is necessary to sustain program success through the fast-paced, ever-changing landscape of health care. Nurse executives engage organizational experts to identify strengths, weaknesses, opportunities, and threats through targeted organizational analyses and deliberate dialogue. These activities focus on the envisioned future state and articulate the path forward through development and implementation of programmatic initiatives. This responsibility requires a sophisticated set of leadership skills and a keen sense of coordination. Such is necessary for the multifaceted approaches that are required to manage the complex nature of nursing practice. A servant leadership style promotes organizational **vision** and communicates the strategic plan to staff. This delicate dance of leading and engaging experts in the process of planning projects and managing programs is an art and a science requiring specialized skills, abilities, and talents.

This chapter provides insight into the required skills and competencies for planning projects and managing programs. The knowledge of subject matter experts for program development and the unique skill set of project managers are a winning combination for actualizing strategic goals of the project and ongoing program management.

Investment in the development of skills and competencies for project planning and ongoing program management is the cornerstone of a successful strategic approach to shaping nursing practice. Academic and practice settings would be well served by understanding the relevance of these principles and are encouraged to provide necessary training and resources to achieve a well-defined desired future state. Nurses are ideally placed to lead and manage projects. They are responsible for managing direct patient care as well as executive decision making. An investment in developing nurses' skill sets will impact not only that nurse, but the organization's ability to meet goals and objectives (O'Neil, Morjikian, Cherner, Hirschorn, & West, 2008).

Core Skill Sets

Managing a project or a program is a balancing act between three general sets of skills: task orientation, management orientation, and leadership orientation. Task orientation is the short-time horizon whereby a project has a distinct beginning, middle, and end. Management orientation focuses on **communication** and interpersonal skills. Leadership orientation is about vision and leveraging one's authority to get the job done (Wagner, 2006). Project management is more readily associated with task orientation as the focus is a singular objective with specific output(s). The implementation of a nursing informatics application such as a computer-based patient handoff system serves as an example. Program management, on the other hand, involves the coordination of multiple projects to create a specific outcome. Examples include reducing medical errors and improving patient safety through the interoperability of multiple nursing informatics applications (Nokes & Kelly, 2008). Project management requires elements of management and leadership orientation. Management and leadership orientation are particularly critical for program management involving more complex governing structures with fundamental changes to the organization as a whole.

A set of skills commonly referred to as "hard skills" apply to task orientation and refer to technical or administrative procedures that are essential to planning, scheduling, and controlling a project. These are distinct from soft skills (also known as people skills) for which the focus is on interpersonal behaviors and involve people management, leadership, and communication styles (Coates, 2006). There are three general hard skills involved in task orientation, which include defining the project, establishing a project management plan, and implementing a control process to monitor progress.

Defining the project is the first step. Stakeholders must agree on the goals, objectives, assumptions, and constraints. Once the project is defined and the desired output has been identified, it is essential to develop a project management plan. This step establishes the overall blueprint for how the desired output will become reality. The path to the desired destination is clearly defined and carefully planned. The appropriate resources must be identified and appropriately utilized. To accomplish this, the project manager must possess skills necessary to develop a project plan that does the following:

1. Revalidates and confirms the project goals and objectives.
2. Identifies the stakeholders, roles and responsibilities, and a schedule of the tasks required.
3. Determines project milestones and criteria for success.

For example, when planning a project to increase patient satisfaction in acute care through improved pain management, patients, families, and treatment teams would be identified as stakeholders. Outlining the cycle of how pain is currently assessed, managed, and monitored would be essential to the improvement process. Each stakeholder's role and responsibility in this process would be identified, as would be the flow of communication and action. Describing the structure, process, and outcomes for the new and improved pain management program would further delineate how this particular project would demonstrate success. Outcomes such as improved patient satisfaction through timely **assessment**, reduced pain scores, and patient's greater sense of autonomy through self-management are examples that may be monitored and of interventions that can be adapted as needed.

Throughout the project's life cycle, it is important to revisit the plan to account for unanticipated issues and to make adjustments accordingly as the project evolves. A control process ensures that projects are on target and the desired results are being achieved. The control process involves monitoring progress and ensuring the project management plan is on the right path towards achieving the desired output. A variety of tools, such as control charts, histograms, and decision trees can be useful when evaluating outcomes. For example, a project developed to reduce wait times in an ambulatory clinic through a kiosk check-in could be measured by a histogram with before and after time series. Analyzing variances between what was planned and what occurred promotes an environment of accountability. A control process accomplishes the following:

1. Establishment of a communication plan to maintain a coordination of efforts among the stakeholders.
2. Identification of criteria for success so that stakeholders have a baseline for tracking progress against expected results.
3. Establishment of a process for continuous and adequate status reports for the agreed-upon tasks.

Once the hard skills have been engaged, application of management and leadership orientation and the applicable soft skills serve as the fuel to drive the project to fruition. For example, skill sets may include visionary leadership, organizational stewardship, flexibility and adaptability, mentorship, and communication. As a visionary leader, consideration would be given to establishing the vision and engaging stakeholders as partners. As a steward of the organization, creating a linkage to related projects and programs is paramount for future success.

Key Components Linking Project Plans to Programs

Effective governance is critical to program success. A poorly articulated management structure, overlapping roles and decision-making authority, and roles filled by the wrong people can prevent a project and/or program from achieving sustained momentum. The system can also be bogged down by endless attempts to achieve consensus on every decision made during the program management process.

Program governance is the aspect of the discipline that creates both the structure and practices to guide the program and obtain senior level leadership involvement, oversight, and authority. Strategically, it encompasses the relationship between the oversight effort and the enterprise's overall business direction. It also defines all the decision-making roles and responsibilities involved in executing the project and overall program effort.

Program management, as compared to project planning, requires a more complex governing structure as it involves fundamental business change and expenditures with significant bottom line impact. In fact, in some instances the outcomes of a particular program can determine whether the enterprise will survive as a viable commercial/government entity. Project management is concerned with the dynamic allocation, utilization, and direction of resources. Within a program, these same responsibilities are assigned to people at different levels in the management hierarchy; the higher the level, the more general the responsibilities. For example, at the microsystem level of the management hierarchy, nurse managers are assigned to the various projects within the overall program. Each nurse manager carries out the management responsibilities described previously.

Program management differs from project management in several fundamental ways. The key difference between a program and a project is the finite nature of a project. Projects have beginning and end dates. When contrasting program and project management, several parameters can be considered. The parameters may include the organization; the alignment of the program and project to the organization; sequencing; and any risk to the overall mission, value, and strategic initiatives. From an organizational perspective, projects are transient and resourced for a limited set of requirements; whereas programs are resourced for longer periods in order to achieve a strategic business objective.

Educating Others to Achieve Project and Program Successes

There is overlap in strategies for educating members of a project team towards the completion of a particular project. This differs from educating future project or program managers. For one, training an individual to complete a task (or set of tasks) as a member of a project team has a finite duration, requiring a more generalized education of the skills needed for the individual to complete the task. The project/program manager in this case can use the key characteristics noted previously to ensure each team member has the resources needed to complete the task(s) assigned. Team members are guided through the process by the project manager, as determined by the type of project team (standard, matrix, or mixed) charged with the task. The standard project team will require higher involvement from the project manager throughout the phases of work, whereas a matrix team can work fairly independently once project tasks have been assigned. The project manager must also ensure that the team is functioning as a team and personality issues do not impede progress.

Teaching future project and program managers whose primary responsibilities will be in either of these roles for an undefined period of time requires a robust set of core skills and competencies and thus a more robust training curriculum. Phase-by-phase strategies that instructors can use, such as the experiential learning activity (ELA), aids the future project manager (Cook & Olson, 2006). ELAs are a form of an accelerated learning activity that enables one to visualize the real-world application of the knowledge being taught. The four phases of the ELA include:

1. Planning—communicating the purpose of the exercise, including objectives, to be reemphasized during the activity.
2. Introduction—providing the instructions to be executed during the activity.
3. Activity—completing the activity (most important in planning for the effectiveness of the whole activity).
4. Feedback—allowing students to reflect and to debrief openly on the important decisions and steps taken during the process.

Accelerated learning techniques and activities such as the ELA assist in helping the learner absorb the intricacies of complex project planning and program management processes that traditional by-the-book education does not permit.

In today's environment of continuous, on-the-go learning, it is also important that educators in project planning and program management utilize all technological resources available to cater to the diversity of their students. The George Washington University, for example, has employed an array of resources since implementing its initial master's program in 1996 that allows not only full-time students, but also professionals, to engage in the topics of program and project management through multiple course tracks (Rad, 2000). Making multiple modes of learning available to those willing to learn increases the chances that the knowledge will be retained.

In educating others in project planning and program management, various strategies and tools can be used to provide a comprehensive learning experience.

The outcome of successful project/program managers and teams requires a good educator and use of practical application experiences matched with theory, flexibility, and innovation in teaching methods.

Case Example

A nursing leadership team that is equipped with well-developed skills and competencies to manage programs with supportive project management principles as described in this chapter will demonstrate an engaged organizational approach to advance nursing practice. Relying on a servant leadership style creates an operational focus that zeros in on meaningful strategic goals to address current and future challenges such as workforce issues that impact effective retention and recruitment initiatives. This example is based on a retention and recruitment goal to support new graduate nurses and a strategic approach to reduce registered nurse turnover rates and improve quality and safety for patients as well as enhanced staff satisfaction.

The nursing leadership team has responsibility to develop and maintain a healthy work environment. As one of the key strategic initiatives, program managers find through published scientific evidence that registered nurse residency programs have a positive impact on quality and safety with concrete findings that the business case describes as solid return on investment. Program managers develop the proposal to pilot a registered nurse residency program that is clearly aligned with overarching organizational priorities. The framework for implementation, communication, and evaluation plans for the pilot is developed by the program managers. Involvement by key stakeholders is designed by the program managers. Program managers work with project managers in parallel to the process described here. Project managers are responsible for working with project team members to fully develop the envisioned pilot. They guide content experts through the process of addressing required elements of implementation, communication, and evaluation plans. The project management skill set offers efficient and comprehensive organization to the many moving parts within this pilot. Efforts are coordinated and integrated under the guidance of project managers working in concert with program managers who have ultimate responsibility for aligning this pilot with other projects related to creating a healthy work environment. Project managers work across various projects as a means to support essential coordination and integration efforts for the program managers. This partnership approach is an essential operating principle for success.

Summary

- Competencies and skills of project planners and program managers are complementary.
- When working in partnership, project and program planning principles strengthen the impact of strategic initiatives.
- Engaging both project and program managers with well-developed skills in an organizational structure facilitates efficient and effective utilization of high-level leadership talent.

Reflection Questions

1. What are the distinctions between project and program management skill sets?
2. What are the advantages of organizing leadership teams to include both project and program and managers?
3. How would you utilize an understanding of competencies and skills of project and program managers to determine the most efficient approach to manage a broad-scoped complex portfolio of responsibilities?

Learning Activity

Invite healthcare administration graduate students to a nursing leadership strategic planning discussion. Assign these students to critique proposed plans for programmatic initiatives and offer suggestions to apply project management principles to the process. Engage the full group in a discussion on pros and cons of a project/program management partnership. Identify potential impact on efficiency and effectiveness of this approach.

References

Coates, D. E. (2006). *People skills training: Are you getting a return on your investment?* Retrieved from http://www.2020insight.net/DOCS4/PeopleSkills.pdf

Cook, L. S., & Olson, J. R. (2006). Index to Journal of Management Education. *Journal of Management Education, 30*(3), 401–524.

Nokes, S., & Kelly, C. (2008). *The definitive guide to project management: The fast track to getting the job done on time and on budget* (2nd ed.). Englewoods Cliffs, NJ: Prentice Hall.

O'Neil, E., Morjikian, R. L., Cherner, D., Hirschorn, C., & West, T. (2008). Developing nursing leaders: An overview of trends and programs. *Journal of Nursing Administration, 38*(4), 178–183.

Rad, P. F. (2000). Project management education through distance learning. *Cost Engineering, 42*(11), 38–40.

Wagner, P. (2006, August). Three skills you need to have for successful project management. *Information Outlook,* 1–5.

FOUR

Team Power and Synergy: Project Planning and Program Management Essentials

■ Sandra E. Walters

■ **Learning Objectives**

1. Identify essential elements of effective teams.
2. Identify and compare the stages of team development.
3. Identify barriers to effectiveness in interdisciplinary teams.
4. Identify multiple strategies for use in managing work.

> "Never doubt that a small group of thoughtful, committed citizens can change the world."
>
> —Margaret Mead

Key Terms

Ad hoc committee

Adjourning

Brainstorming

Collaborating

Forming

Interdisciplinary team

Multidisciplinary team

Nominal grouping

Norming

Performing

Program management

Project planning

SBAR communication

Storming

Synergy

Task force

Team

Roles

Advocate

Communicator

Decision maker

Integrator

Leader

Risk anticipator

Professional Values

Altruism

Evidence-based practice

Integrity

Patient-centric care

Quality

Social justice

Core Competencies

Appreciative inquiry

Assessment

Coordination

Critical thinking

Design

Emotional intelligence

Health promotion

Interpersonal influence

Leadership

Management

Resource management

Risk reduction

Systems thinking

Introduction

There are times when one single individual may possess the knowledge, skills, and abilities to bring about changes in a healthcare system that result in the improvement of care delivery. Singular skills are important, yet to get true buy-in, stakeholder participation is critical. The implementation of any initiative from **project planning** and **program management** can be facilitated through the work of **teams**, and thus it is essential to understand how to maximize the effectiveness of using a team approach.

Essential Elements of Teams

The word *team* has evolved from the original Old English word, *teme*, which indicated lineage, to a later term that referred to two or more animals harnessed to a single vehicle, to its present-day use, which includes several persons associated by work or activity (Merriam-Webster, 2010). Whether one is speaking about football, baseball, corporations, departments, or offices, the word *team* often implies that members of a group are all working toward a common goal or purpose. An examination of the concept of teams in the healthcare literature reveals the frequent use of the terms *interdisciplinary* and *multidisciplinary* in referring to the composition of the teams. Careful examination shows these terms are often used interchangeably, although there is a difference and the distinction is important.

One widely used definition of **interdisciplinary team** was put forth by Drinka and Clark (2000), who defined it as individuals working together in a group to solve problems too complex to be addressed by one discipline or multiple disciplines acting in sequence. Inherent in this definition of the interdisciplinary team is that individuals have diversity in training and in their backgrounds, and that they come together collaboratively in formal or informal structures. The use of individuals who come together from different disciplines allows the team to capitalize on the variations in the approach to problems, provides opportunities for learning about overlapping roles, and accounts for power differences within the organization while establishing the goals and mission of the team.

Similarly, a **multidisciplinary team** also includes professionals from a range of disciplines working together to solve a problem such as would be presented by the complex healthcare needs of a patient with multiple medical issues (Von Gunten, Ferris, Portenoy, & Glajchen, 2001). Underlying the concept of the multidisciplinary team is that each discipline performs its functions in a sequential manner rather than as a member of an interacting and **collaborating** group, and the goals of each discipline may be established separately from those of the other members of the group (Mitchell, Tieman, & Shelby-James, 2008).

To illustrate the difference between an interdisciplinary team and multidisciplinary team, it is useful to examine the fictional case of patient Imogene Withers (**Box 4-1**).

Box 4-1 Case Study

Mrs. Imogene Withers is an 82-year-old widow admitted to her local hospital following a fall at the local grocery store. On admission, she was found to have a hip fracture and low serum glucose and was noted to live alone. After her hip-replacement surgery, a multidisciplinary discharge planning conference was held on the unit to discuss the patient's potential for discharge. The nurse, surgeon, an internal medicine doctor, physical therapist, social worker, dietitian, and occupational therapist were in attendance. When discussing Mrs. Withers, the surgeon indicated the fracture was healing slowly and he was concerned regarding the patient's ability to ambulate. The physical therapist and occupational therapist reported each had been treating the patient and concurred that her progress had been slower than expected and that she would require more extensive rehabilitation. The dietitian indicated she could evaluate the patient's nutritional status to determine if she had sufficient nutrients to promote healing. The medical doctor indicated Mrs. Withers's hypoglycemia had been attributed to a lack of nutritional intake but that subsequent laboratory tests were within normal limits and no further follow-up for this was needed. The team made the decision to place Ms. Withers in a rehabilitation unit until sufficient progress was made to discharge the patient to her home. Each member of the multidisciplinary team documented his or her recommendations for follow-up care in the patient record.

Mrs. Withers's transfer to the rehabilitation unit was completed and was followed by a request from her nurse to assemble an interdisciplinary team to establish the goals of her care. In addition to Mrs. Withers, the nurse, an internal medicine doctor, a physical therapist, a social worker, a dietitian, and an occupational therapist were in attendance. Following discussion with Mrs. Withers, it was determined that the team would seek to maximize Mrs. Withers's quality of life and safety. The social worker agreed to explore options for Mrs. Withers's living arrangements once she went home and she arranged to meet with the therapists to determine how to address Mrs. Withers's limitations for living alone. Additionally, the team determined pain and fatigue were deterring Mrs. Withers from participating fully in her therapy, and thus plans were made to provide pain medication prior to therapy and to allow sufficient rest periods between activities. Subsequently, each member of the team determined how he or she could contribute to enhancing Mrs. Withers's quality of life and while addressing her safety requirements. When all the plans were finalized, the nurse documented the interdisciplinary team member proceedings including the plan of care, expected outcomes, and follow-up plans.

Upon review of the case presented on the care of Mrs. Withers, it should be noted that the multidisciplinary approach presents the work of several disciplines with each focusing on its goals for the patient. By contrast, the interdisciplinary approach brings together multiple disciplines, but the goal is one common goal for all disciplines, with everyone assuming complementary roles and working together toward the same ends. In effect, each discipline loses its separate identity and its goals become those of the team (Von Gunten et al., 2001).

Applying concepts of team energy to project management, this seamless approach underscores the need for continuity and flow. In addition to interdisciplinary and multidisciplinary teams, other types of groups that can be formed for problem-solving initiatives are those of **task forces** and **ad hoc committees**. Task forces are groups of individuals who come together for the purpose of completing a given assignment or goal within defined time limits. In similar manner, an ad hoc committee is one formed temporarily to address a specific issue within a specific time frame but is additionally created from a larger grouping or committee (American Heritage Dictionary, 2009). Because of the complexity of the healthcare system, it is assumed that task forces and ad hoc committees will be comprised of individuals from a variety of disciplines, and thus the task forces and ad hoc committees will possess characteristics similar to those of the interdisciplinary teams.

Stages in Team Development

One of the advantages of teams has been identified as providing staff from multiple departments opportunities to resolve operational issues by bringing their knowledge of what needs to be fixed together with a mechanism to collaborate and take actions (Studer, 2003). This advantage is believed to be the result of **synergy**, which is the phenomenon that occurs when the whole is greater than the sum of its parts as happens with teamwork (Sholtes, 2010). Whether the teams are composed of multiple professionals functioning as a team within one organization or of professionals from multiple organizations, the development of the team is believed to undergo similar stages during the course of work. Four stages of team synergy were identified by Bruce Tuckman in 1965 as including **forming**, **storming**, **norming**, and **performing**, with a fifth stage, **adjourning**, identified in 1977 (Tuckman, 2001).

During forming, the team is assembled, and each member is initially focused on his/her own objectives. Orientation to the tasks or team goals takes place during this phase, and team members often engage in behaviors that test the group dynamics (Tuckman, 2001). Team members' emotional response may vary widely from pride in their selection for the team to apprehension regarding the work ahead (Sholtes, 2010). As the orientation is completed and the tasks and requirements become evident, resistance to the group influence emerges and intragroup conflict may arise, which indicates the team is storming (Tuckman, 2001). During this stage, team members have low levels of trust and often display anger and resentment. While turf battles may ensue, the foundations for trust and respect may be developed during this stage based on how conflicts are resolved. During the norming phase that follows, group cohesiveness develops, and members adjust to their roles in the team (Tuckman, 2001). Open communication during this phase facilitates constructive discussions and the sharing of personal insights (Sholtes, 2010). As the team members bind together around their common goals, the work phase of the team begins and productivity increases rapidly during the performing stage (Tuckman, 2001). Team synergy becomes evident as member roles become flexible and the focus shifts to the tasks at hand. Members will display team loyalty, will be able to capitalize on individual strengths, and will support team efforts. As tasks are completed and the outcomes of the work lead to self-evaluation by the team and its members, the adjourning phase is reached and may lead to sadness and mourning as members face the completion of the goals and group tasks (Tuckman, 2001). A summary of Tuckman's stages of team development is presented in **Table 4-1**.

It should be noted that while Tuckman's model suggests a linear relationship among the phases of team synergy formation, the stages may not occur sequentially

Table 4-1 Tuckman's Stages of Team Development

Stage	Member Dynamics	Task Orientation
1. Forming	Members focus on their goals	Team established
	Group dynamics are tested	Orientation of team members
	Pride or apprehension evident	
2. Storming	Resistance to group goals	Emotional response to tasks
	Conflicts often evident	
	Trust in group is low	Turf wars possible
3. Norming	Trust is established	Role adjustment occurs
	Open communication allowed	
	Ideas shared and accepted	
4. Performing	Team loyalty evident	Greatest productivity
	Use of member strengths	Focus is on tasks and goals
	Positive attitudes evident	
5. Adjourning	Evaluation of outcomes	Team dissolved or transformed
	Sadness or mourning may begin as tasks are completed	

and may be repeated or interrupted at any point in time. Unexpected occurrences, such as the introduction of a new team member, may disrupt established team dynamics and may shift the team to either an earlier or later stage (Tuckman, 2001).

Barriers to Effectiveness in Interdisciplinary Teams

Progression through the stages of team development as identified by Tuckman requires that the team achieve efficiency at each stage. Lencioni (2002) identified barriers to effectiveness at each stage that undermine the effectiveness of teams and cause them to fail in their endeavors. Problems he identified among team members included an inability to trust or have reliance on others, fear of conflict, lack of commitment, having low standards such that accountability is avoided, and inattention to the results of the team and instead a focus on individual achievement.

Addressing each of the barriers identified by Lencioni (2002) is possible through effective leadership. To begin with, the responsibility of a program planner or project manager is to assist team members in developing trust by demonstrating reliance on the team as a means of overcoming the limitation in the knowledge, skills, or abilities of any individual team members. One means to achieve this is through a willingness to demonstrate vulnerability. The second limitation, that of fearing conflict, requires that team leaders support constructive debates and demonstrate the ability to manage it by establishing group norms for dealing with issues in a manner that is respectful of all team members. With a lack of commitment, the underlying problem is a lack of decision-making capacity by the team such that individuals seek consensus instead of achieving a clear position on issues. This can be resolved through inclusion of all points of view in making decisions. Similarly, a lack of accountability can be countered by assisting the team to focus on goals, continually tracking team progress, and communicating frequently with the team through meetings and status reports. Finally, inattention to the results of the team can be minimized through the selection of measures that clearly define success for the team effort and the development of a tracking mechanism to monitor team progress. Success and failures must be equally shared within the team and used to reinforce progress to goals.

In addition to the barriers identified by Lencioni (2002), Atwal and Caldwell (2006) conducted a study of nurses' perception regarding multidisciplinary teamwork and identified barriers that hinder teamwork as including the following:

- Different perceptions of teamwork are held by nurses compared with other members of the team.
- A difference in the level of skills required for team members to function within teams is often present.
- Disciplines lack equal power within teams with medical power being dominant.

Their findings suggest that educators and nursing managers should focus on developing staff member abilities to function within teams, and the team skills must include an understanding of the nurse's role as well as those of other disciplines.

Multiple barriers to efficient team functioning in healthcare settings have been identified and are often presented as communication obstacles that are listed in **Box 4-2** (Agency for Healthcare Research and Quality, 2008; O'Daniel & Rosenstein, 2008).

The development of cooperative agendas can ameliorate the impact of communication barriers and can be facilitated by the fact that healthcare team members generally share the value of meeting the needs of patients or clients (O'Daniel & Rosenstein, 2008).

Box 4-2 Communication Obstacles to Team Effectiveness

Gender differences
Distraction (cellular phones, pagers)
Fatigue
Excessive workload
Time constraints
Hierarchical relationships
Information silos
Differences in accountability, compensation, and rewards
Cultural and ethnic differences
Historical professional rivalries
Language and terminology differences
Disruptive behaviors, aggression

Strategies for Work Management

The use of standardized communication tools to support teamwork in complexity of the healthcare environment has been explored in the literature as a means of improving decision making and increasing safety (O'Daniel & Rosenstein, 2008). Strategies include the use of techniques such as **brainstorming, nominal grouping, and SBAR communication.**

Brainstorming sessions are used to generate a large number of ideas through interaction among team members. In this strategy, the objective of the brainstorming is established and is often directly related to the team goals. One individual is selected to record ideas (generally on a board or flip chart) to avoid duplications. Individuals in the group then call out ideas in turn with the process continuing until no further ideas emerge. The essential rules of brainstorming are that everyone participates and that no discussion, critique, or evaluation of the ideas takes place during the session. Following the creative thinking session, each is clarified to facilitate subsequent discussion of its feasibility.

In similar manner, the nominal group process begins with the establishment of an objective but proceeds with each member generating his or her own list of possible solutions. When sufficient time has been allowed, members take turns calling out their ideas to the group. As with the brainstorming session, ideas are not discussed until all have been presented. Once the list of ideas is complete, clarification follows as with the brainstorming session.

Once ideas are generated using brainstorming or nominal group processes, the team proceeds to decrease the list by such mechanisms as voting to eliminate ideas that are not feasible, identifying items that may be readily implemented (low-hanging fruit), and rank ordering related alternatives. Rank ordering can be accomplished by having individual team members rank each idea and then calculating average scores for each idea to determine the degree of agreement amongst team members. Clarification and discussion of the strengths, weaknesses, opportunities, and threats of each idea can be undertaken by the team and is referred to as a SWOT analysis. Additionally, an affinity diagram, in which ideas are written on cards and placed randomly on a table or chart, can be generated. Like or related ideas are then placed together by group members working silently. When cards are no longer being moved, the group then discusses the ideas and generates a title for each group. Each method is useful in exploring alternative plans of action towards goal attainment.

An additional strategy, that of SBAR communication, was developed at Kaiser Permanente and is among the techniques useful in teamwork for communicating essential information using a standardized format. In this strategy, communication is provided using the format of situation, background, assessment, and recommendation (SBAR). To begin with, the situation is outlined using a brief summary of what is going on. This is followed by background information about the clinical situation or the context of the issue. The assessment component presents a statement of what the individual has identified as the problem and is followed by a recommendation of what corrective action is needed. Originally developed to facilitate communication between nurses and physicians, the use of a standardized format within team communication dynamics provides a succinct method of communicating information rapidly.

The work of a team to improve processes can be both challenging and rewarding. Effective leadership is facilitated through the use of structures and tools to ensure participation by all members of the team.

Summary

- Implementation of any initiative from project planning and program management can be facilitated through the work of teams.
- Five stages of team synergy are forming, storming, norming, performing, and adjourning.
- Problems in team development include inability to trust, fear of conflict, lack of commitment, low standards, and inattention to results.
- Multiple strategies may be used to increase the effectiveness of teamwork and include the use of brainstorming, nominal group processes, affinity diagrams, SWOT analyses, and the use of SBAR communication techniques.

Reflection Questions

1. During a period of prolonged emergency leave by the chairperson of the patient safety committee, hospital administrators have requested you assume responsibility for decreasing the number of patient falls in the rehabilitation unit. Upon arriving at the meeting of the patient falls committee, you note members of the rehabilitation medicine teams are sitting together apart from the rest of the group. As the meeting begins, you note they are whispering to each other and are not contributing to the discussions.

   Identify the stage of team development. Identify multiple strategies to use in moving the group forward in achieving the goals of reducing patient falls.

2. The medical unit at a local hospital has identified the need to convene an interdisciplinary team to facilitate intrafacility transfers. Identify what disciplines you would include in the team. Determine what communication norms would be useful to enhance the work of the team.

Learning Activities

1. Identify what committees, teams, or task forces are in place at your local healthcare facility. Attend their meetings and use Tuckman's model to determine what stage of development each team is in.

2. Analyze communication strategies in use during a departmental meeting. Compare this to the communication strategies in use during an interdisciplinary team meeting. What similarities or differences exist? Identify effective strategies in use, potential barriers to communication, and mechanisms for their elimination.

References

Agency for Healthcare Research and Quality. (2008). *TeamSTEPPS rapid response systems module: Instructor's materials*. Retrieved from http://www.ahrq.gov/info/customer.htm

American Heritage Dictionary of the English Language (4th ed.). (2009). New York: Houghton Mifflin Company.

Atwal, A., & Caldwell, C. (2006). Nurses' perceptions of multidisciplinary team work in acute health-care. *International Journal of Nursing Practice, 12*(6), 359–365.

Drinka, T. J. K., & Clark, P. G. (2000). *Health care teamwork: Interdisciplinary practice & teaching*. Westport, CT: Greenwood Publishing Group.

Lencioni, P. M. (2002). *The five dysfunctions of a team: A leadership fable*. San Francisco: Jossey-Bass.

Merriam-Webster. (2010). Team. In *Merriam-Webster online dictionary*. Retrieved from http://www.merriam-webster.com/dictionary/team

Mitchell, G. K., Tieman, J. J., & Shelby-James, T. M. (2008). Multidisciplinary care planning and teamwork in primary care. *Medical Journal of Australia, 188*(8), 63.

O'Daniel, M., & Rosenstein, A. H. (2008). Professional communication and team collaboration. In R. G. Hughes (Ed.), *Patient safety and quality: An evidence-based handbook for nurses* (Vol. 2). Rockville, MD: Agency for Healthcare Research and Quality.

Sholtes, P. R. (2010). *Team dynamics*. Retrieved from http://www.cls.utk.edu/pdf/ls/Week3_Lesson17.pdf

Studer, Q. (2003). *Hardwiring excellence: Purpose, worthwhile work, making a difference*. Gulf Breeze, FL: Fire Starter Publishing.

Tuckman, B. W. (2001). Development sequence in small groups. *Group Facilitation: A Research and Applications Journal, 3*, 66–81.

Von Gunten, C. F., Ferris F. D., Portenoy, R. K., & Glajchen, M. (Eds.). (2001). *CAPC manual: How to establish a palliative care program*. New York: Center to Advance Palliative Care.

FIVE

Planning a Project for Implementation

■ Catherine Dearman and Debra Davis

■ Learning Objectives

1. Discuss the primary steps in planning a sustainable project.
2. Describe the life cycle of a project plan.
3. Consider a clinical micro, meso, and macrosystem model as a tool for diagnosing a system's needs.
4. Identify the types of project risks, how to assess for risks, and address them.
5. Describe stakeholders' role in supporting a project and program.
6. Explain how to build the case for a sustainable project.

> "A good solution solves more than one problem."
>
> —Wendell Berry

Key Terms

Clinical micro, meso,
  or macrosystems

Risk management

Stakeholders

Roles

Communicator

Decision maker

Information manager

Integrator

Leader

Risk anticipator

Professional Values

Altruism

Integrity

Social justice

Core Competencies

Assessment

Critical thinking/
  appreciative inquiry

Design

Emotional intelligence

Interpersonal influence

Leadership

Management and coordination

Risk reduction

System thinking

Introduction

The purpose of this chapter is to facilitate your success when undertaking projects in a variety of clinical and work environments. Lewis stated that work done in organizations could be described as a project. If you have ever been involved in any phase of instituting a new policy or developing a new protocol in your healthcare facility, you have engaged in some aspect of project planning and/or management.

Project management has the following two major components: determining what is to be done and establishing how it will be accomplished. Both of these major components are introduced to stakeholders as a part of a comprehensive project plan, which most authors agree is essential to the actual accomplishment of desired outcomes. Most people would say that a good outcome is predicated on good planning. Theoretically, if the plan is sound and the execution follows the plan, success is virtually guaranteed. Why, then, do so many projects fail? One reason may be the lack of a comprehensive, detailed plan that accounts for contingencies or the unexpected.

Major aspects of planning a project will be addressed in this chapter, including assessing the environment; establishing the need and evidentiary basis underlying the change; developing a strategy for accomplishing the plan, which includes identifying alternative solutions and selecting the appropriate one for the environment; and, finally, projecting desired/expected outcomes. All project team members must be on the same page with regard to the issues and desired outcomes in order for planning to be effective and inclusive. Without such careful planning, it can truly be a one-step-forward-and-two-steps-backward process.

Assessing the Environment

As a general rule, there is more than one way to accomplish any project. The challenge is to identify the best strategy for a particular environment and situation. A comprehensive needs assessment involves these two main areas: an assessment of strengths, weaknesses, opportunities, and threats (a SWOT analysis), and a gap analysis. A needs assessment can take many forms, dependent upon the type of unit, system, or organization being assessed, but it typically involves an objective review of internal processes and personnel. During a SWOT analysis, all aspects of the system are fully examined from a **clinical micro, meso, or macrosystem** perspective. The SWOT analysis will assist the project manager and team in identifying internal and external aspects that may positively or negatively affect the project. An example follows.

In a regular quarterly review, the no-show rate of an outpatient cardiovascular catheterization lab was found to be 20% higher than in the previous three quarters of the year. In an effort to understand the data before her annual report to administration was due, the unit manager conducted a needs assessment. She reviewed patient scheduling processes, interviewed physicians and staff to determine their perspectives, and determined the presumed cause of the rise in no shows to the unit to be a new staff member who had assumed responsibility for scheduling patients without fully understanding the complex nature of the cardiovascular lab's operation. The unit manager developed a comprehensive plan to educate the new staff member, fully orient her to all aspects of patient scheduling, and, hopefully, eliminate the problem. However, over the next few weeks, it became evident that the number of no shows actually rose rather than fell. Hospital administrators became aware of the issue and asked for a comprehensive assessment of the situation. The clinical nurse leader for outpatient services was tasked with completing the needs assessment. In the clinical nurse leader's SWOT analysis, she determined that the issue was not within the system but outside it. Over the past several weeks, the city had been working on drainage lines in the neighborhood, causing a diversion in the traffic pattern. The city transit service could no longer access the parking lot closest to the outpatient cardiovascular lab, causing patients to have to walk around the building, a far greater distance. Once the traffic diversion was corrected, the no-show rate returned to a very reasonable 3%. The clinical nurse leader in this example performed a comprehensive assessment of the situation using a new lens and identified the external threat to full functioning of the lab.

A full SWOT assessment of the system assists the team in developing strategies to deal with known forces, both internal and external, and to anticipate others. In a SWOT analysis, each of the elements must be thoroughly analyzed, clearly communicated to all stakeholders, and planned for within distinct limits. Only through accounting for the processes and mechanisms currently occurring within a system can one determine where gaps exist. The project plan is typically directed at resolving one or more gaps. In the case study above, the unit manager conducted a partial analysis, not a comprehensive one.

A gap analysis is a critical step in establishing both the problem and the evidence to support the need for the project. A gap analysis is dependent upon identification of existing resources, politics, and culture within the environment. The strategy to deal with the items identified in the SWOT and gap analyses is up to the project team, facilitated by the project manager. Decisions will need to be made regarding factors triggering additions or changes to be made in the plan, factors that can be ignored or bypassed or steps taken to neutralize any issues, providing of course that the issues are known. For example, in preparing for a revision of patient admission processes, the project team analyzes current resources. The team discovers an individual on staff who has extensive skills, talent, and experience in patient admissions. This previously overlooked individual could play an integral role in the project, reducing the overall costs while facilitating sustainability. The identification of this individual casts new light on the project and causes a redirection of effort, saving financial and other resources. In this case, the perceived gap did not exist.

In another example, the team considers external forces that may impact the initiation of a new urgent clinic to alleviate overuse of the emergency department. The team discovers that other clinics in the area have recently expanded services to address the issue. This duplication of services offered elsewhere within the community causes opposition from **stakeholders** and builds political fallout. The clinic project is reviewed and revised to more comprehensively meet the need without duplicating services already available in the community. The network of care services that results is used as a national model of integration of care. Again, a comprehensive SWOT and gap analysis saved resources and enhanced sustainability of the projects.

Developing the Strategy

Strategy is the overall approach to the project and generally encompasses identifying alternative solutions to a problem and, through a process of elimination, selecting the appropriate one for the environment or situation. In the case of planning a project, the project manager must balance all variables and alternatives and choose the best path while meeting the budget allocation, providing the best quality outcome, meeting performance measures, and maintaining scope all within the allotted time frame for project completion.

Organizations deal with developing planning process strategies in a variety of ways. While some agencies hire consultants from outside the organization to develop project plans, generally speaking, most projects require the early involvement of individuals who understand the organizational culture and dynamics. Knowing the internal processes within an organization informs development of sustainable strategies for change. Within the SWOT analysis, each layer of the system is addressed: micro, meso, and macro for facilitators and barriers to project completion. A project such as decreasing the time between a patient's call bell alarming and a response is appropriate for clinical nurse leaders, specifically occurring at the micro, or unit, level. While a meso-level project addresses communication between units, a doctor of nursing practice nurse executive student would be better equipped given his or her skills in negotiation and persuasion. A meso project may take the form of decreasing the wait times in the emergency department for a transfer to a medical surgical unit. Such a project may entail working with the emergency department staff and the nursing unit, and as well as the transport, housekeeping, and admitting departments. Meso-level projects are of greater complexity. Macro-level projects are typically the most complex of all and reflect the needs of the entire system. A career ladder program is an example of a macro project affecting an entire facility. Another example may be the implementation of an electronic health record for a health system. Something on that order is typically considered global enough to be seen as a macro project—it impacts all aspects of the organization.

Multiple alternatives may exist in a given environment to accomplish project goals, in which case a process of ranking or prioritizing those alternatives will be needed. Stratifying options may sometimes be a preliminary step to ranking them. Project planners need to assure that they have identified all viable solutions to the problem or gap in service. Developing the strategy, however, does not include significant details about each alternative, but rather it outlines the options in general terms and conditions. Enough information is needed in this phase to compare alternatives; more detailed planning will come later.

Consider the situation of a husband who has forgotten his anniversary until the very last minute. His forgetfulness has been a problem in the past; he must derive a solution that does not point out his lapse in memory. As he considers his approach, he determines that he has the following three acceptable alternatives: flowers, dinner out, or jewelry; all are readily available at the last minute. While all of the alternatives are possibilities, only the person directly involved and who knows all the internal and external forces at work can select the appropriate one. The husband knows that his wife will rapidly determine that flowers are a last-minute gift since he has used this strategy on prior occasions. He immediately rules them out. Dinner out would be easier to schedule and could be a surprise but cost may be a factor and he knows that his wife has been visiting the gym 5 days a week to lose 20 pounds. He is unsure of dinner as a viable option. On the other hand, the jewelry store he passes on his way home each day is open late and they gift wrap! While jewelry was the most expensive option, the associated risks were less, causing it to be the best-fitting alternative. As you can see, while all gifts were viable alternatives in this case, only the person directly involved can order or structure those alternatives and select the best one.

Once alternatives are identified, the project manager leads the team in prioritization and selection of the best one for the current situation. The role of the project manager is essential to the planning process—he/she is the facilitator of the entire project. According to Rettig and Simons (1993), "A good project manager is a remover of obstacles and a provider of resources" (p. 45). The project manager is responsible for setting goals, defining objectives, and delineating strategies for project accomplishment. Aspects of the plan must account for the timeline for implementation with acceptable variations, set thresholds for achievement so that milestones can be accomplished, and assess the agreement of project tasks with available resources.

Project management is far more than simply scheduling the tasks to be performed. Much of project management is in the details associated with the process of how it is to be done. Project management is, to a large extent, process management. The extent to which the project flows smoothly will be determined by the skill of the project manager.

The project manager works collaboratively; planning for the work is best done by the people who do the work. Inclusion facilitates buy-in and sustainability. The project manager works collectively with team members to accomplish the task at hand. It is generally not wise to plan a project and simply deliver it to the site. It is important that engagement be at each level of decision making. Collaboration across organizational stakeholders requires communication, commitment, accountability, and continuity" (McElmurry et al., 2009). Support for a project comes from all aspects of the organization. There is the expectation that all stakeholders (sponsors, decision makers, and leaders) will be committed to the success of the project. Project success is more likely when the project is aligned with the goals and needs of the organization and system it will impact.

Planning for Desired/Expected Outcomes

Planning for implementation is more structured planning than previously described in "Developing the Strategy." The project team and the project manager consider alternatives and prioritize them. All aspects of the selected alternative are mapped and projected. The basic idea behind planning for implementation is identifying and reinforcing the critical capabilities or capacities of the project. Without planning for implementation, essential aspects of the environment, the options, and the personnel might not be considered, possibly causing significant weakness in the plan itself.

Planning for implementation requires that essential questions be asked and answered. Who will do it? When will it be done? What is needed to accomplish the task? How will it be done, and how much cost is involved with regard to time, money, and other resources? Some may say that small projects do not need to address all these aspects, especially if the project director is assuming all the costs and will do the work. Successful project planning, however, is predicated on knowing or at least being able to predict the answers to the who, when, what, and how questions.

The significance of collaboration and communication with stakeholders cannot be understated.

> The leadership team in any organization sets the tone and expectations for the rest of the employees. Therefore, it is important to involve organizational stakeholders from the beginning, provide intermittent progress checks, responsive to concerns, and address risks throughout implementation. (McElmurry et al., 2009)

Several common mistakes associated with the planning for implementation phase of any project can be identified. Mistakes might include having too specific a plan that does not allow flexibility in dealing with an unexpected finding; having a plan that does not involve the people who must do the work; and failure to plan for risks. The first step in detailing an implementation plan is identifying the essential elements. What must be done? Who will perform each task? How long will each task take? What material, supplies, and equipment are required to complete the task? How much will each task cost? An example of an implementation plan is depicted in **Figure 5-1** using a project entitled, Detailing a Car. In this example, the first phase is outlining all aspects of the work to be done such as washing the car body, vacuuming, polishing hard/flat surfaces inside the car, cleaning tires, cleaning glass, preparing the equipment, waxing and buffing, and fine detail work. What you note in the first phase of the plan is that there is no order to the tasks; they are simply listed. The purpose of listing all aspects of the work to be done is to prevent overlooking one or more aspects until the work is actually under way. After all, nothing is worse than preparing to mow the grass and realizing that you loaned the lawn mower to your neighbor who is out of town for the next 2 weeks.

The next phase of planning for implementation is to order the tasks. Some ordering is relatively logical. For example, one would assume that preparing the equipment would precede use of the equipment. The work plan should be developed by those actually doing the work; all work plan development should occur prior to scheduling the tasks to be completed or allocating resources to the project.

Figure 5-1   Detailing a car.

Phase I: Beginning the Process

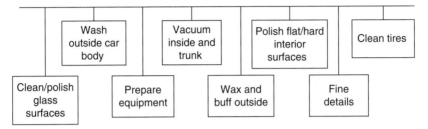

Phase II: Moving into Action

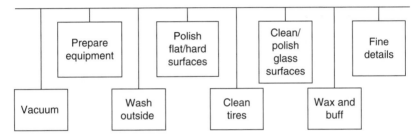

Define who will do each task, how long each task will take, and milestones.
*Example:
   Vacuum
      Car seats (10)
      Door (5)
      Floor mats (10)
      Floor (15)
      Trunk (10)

Involvement of those who will do the work expedites project implementation and achievement of aims; direct knowledge of the work situation and how rapidly tasks can be accomplished can expedite the project's conclusion.

The work plan is detailed enough to provide structure to the project. Too much analysis of the aspects will lead to overkill and negatively impact the energy of the team. A project work plan addresses the four typical constraints that exist in any project implementation: what will be done and who will do the work (scope of the project); how long will the project take (project timeline); what materials and supplies are needed to complete the project and how much each task will cost (cost of project); and the level to which the project will be completed (performance criteria). Some refer to this aspect as "deliverables." Your deliverable(s) will be also be a part of the business plan for the project. An important part of this plan is how success is gauged from project outcomes. What are measurable outcomes that evidence success? The performance criteria developed reflect values of the organization and are quantifiable to demonstrate the value added to the organization. Having quantifiable outcomes as performance criteria facilitates sustainability.

Scheduling the project will be addressed in Chapter 7, "Implementing a Project." The remainder of this chapter will focus on maintaining communication to all stakeholders and damage control—better known as **risk management**.

Planning Communication

An alliance or partnership to complete a project includes stakeholders on both sides of the issue and is predicated on an agreement to conduct the project. Some may think that a small project does not require a basic agreement between parties. However, lack of stipulations regarding product outcome may result in long-term damage to professional relationships. A basic agreement is necessary to ensure that all parties involved clearly understand their responsibilities, including resources to be provided and ownership of any products produced from the project.

Central to project planning is a basic understanding between the organization and group providing the service and the organization or persons receiving or requesting the service. This agreement is comprehensive, allowing full expression of the project itself while being loose enough to allow flexibility in approaches. The agreement includes a thorough description of the project, a list of team members— actual or anticipated—along with their planned contributions to the project, the level of responsibility within the phases of the project, and expected outcomes. The agreement addresses the scope of the project and actions included and also those possibly not anticipated. The agreement is formalized and signed by all parties to aid in clear communication and assignment of responsibility. The agreement will structure team and organizational communication, providing a means of documenting progress toward goal achievement.

Interpersonal skills and effective communication are critical to the project manager role. Projects are people oriented. Project personnel include members of the project team and stakeholders in the project's environment. Winning the support of stakeholders is essential to project sustainability. A strategy for winning support is knowing the stakeholders' areas of interest and demonstrating how the project addresses these interests. For example, structuring a presentation for the nursing staff that focuses on how the project will result in more efficient use of their time rather than being just one more thing they must accomplish during their busy day is more likely to garner support and interest in the project. Finally, people are more likely to respond positively to ideas if there is reciprocal trust and respect between all parties. Excellent communication skills and relating well to others are essential aspects for the project manager.

The organizational representative is also responsible for sending clear and unambiguous information to the project manager. The project manager is responsible for receiving data and factoring this information into project plans. Financial and time overruns, changes in protocol or policy, etc., are common in project management, especially given the fact that most projects occur over several months to years. Change is a necessary consideration of the process—another reason that a contract or agreement between parties is essential.

Planning Risk Management Strategies

Murphy's law indicates that there is a greater probability that things will accidentally go wrong than there is that they will accidentally go right. A risk is anything that may happen that could affect schedule, costs, quality, or scope of work. Risk management is contingency planning and involves careful analysis of what could potentially go wrong and what might be done to prevent the risk or to successfully manage a situation. The careful project manager recognizes that risks are inherent in projects, anticipates them, and works closely with stakeholders in devising ways to overcome challenges, all while preserving continuing opportunities.

A team brainstorming session that asks, "What could happen?" will be beneficial to anticipate what could go wrong in each stage of the plan. Quantifying risk by projecting probability and impact is also important to the planning phase. A part of quantifying the risk is recognizing when it can be ignored or bypassed. Developing a contingency plan to deal with those risks that cannot be ignored or bypassed further enhance project success and sustainability. The project manager skilled in guiding the team through risk assessment and management processes is more likely to ensure team members are versed in appropriate actions to take to identify and manage risks.

Summary

- Planning is critical to a successful project.
- A needs assessment will identify what is in the environment as well as gaps in service.
- Stakeholders must be involved and kept informed at all steps along the way.
- Environmental assessment must account for all levels in a system—micro, meso, and macro.
- Developing a strategy is more than listing tasks to be performed.
- Communicate, communicate, communicate.
- Developing a graphic work flow will help the project team to visualize alternatives and refine time, costs, scope, and performance measures.
- A project manager is a remover of obstacles and a provider of resources.
- Determine all alternatives prior to selecting a course of action and certainly before scheduling project tasks.
- Prioritize all aspects of the project plan to assure that work progresses in a logical manner.
- Account for risks and threats to project.
- Develop a risk management plan to address risks to a project.
- Plan for implementation.
- Allocate sufficient resources to the project.
- Revisit the plan, refine and revise as necessary to keep the project on track.

Reflection Questions

1. As a project manager, what do you think would be an important first step in organizing a team to approach a project?
2. You encounter an unexpected risk to successful implementation of your project. How will you address this risk? What might you have done to prevent the risk?
3. What are some planning strategies that you should consider to assist your appeal to stakeholders?
4. Are there actions that you can take to be more effective in your communication and interpersonal skills?

References

Lewis, J. P. (2005). *Project planning, scheduling, and control.* New York: McGraw-Hill.

McElmurry, B. J., McCreary, L. L., Park, C. G., Ramos, L., Martinez, E., Parikh, R., et al. (2009). Implementation, outcomes, and lessons learned from a collaborative primary health care program to improve diabetes care among urban Latino populations. *Health Promotion Practice, 10*(2), 293–302.

Retting, M., & Simons, G. (1993). A project planning and development process for small teams. *Communication of the ACM, 36,* 45–55.

SIX

The Clinical Needs Assessment: Foundations for Application

■ James L. Harris, Linda Roussel, and Catherine Dearman

■ **Learning Objectives**

1. Identify the primary components of a clinical needs assessment.
2. List the steps to take when completing a needs assessment.
3. Identify the steps for completing an institutional review board submission.
4. Compare a clinical needs assessment and a community needs assessment.

"Where is the wisdom we have lost in knowledge? Where is the knowledge we have lost in information?"

—T. S. Elliot

Key Terms

Clinical needs assessment

Community needs assessment

Institutional review board

Value

Roles

Advocate

Communicator

Decision maker

Designer

Risk anticipator

Professional Values

Integrity

Quality

Core Competencies

Advocacy

Analyzing

Assessment

Communication

Coordination

Design

Development

Management

Introduction

The identification of a need is the cornerstone for project planning when an organization is starting a new clinical program or a community is considering enhancing existing services. Determining in advance what is needed helps in the identification of whether or not to pursue a proposed project (Loo, 2003). Organizations conduct a **clinical needs assessment** and often a SWOT analysis that guide decisions and subsequent project and program activities. Foundational to conducting a clinical needs assessment is the consideration of how the information will be used and if it can be used to improve community services.

If plans include disseminating the findings outside of the organization/area, **institutional review board** (IRB) approval is required. This chapter identifies what a clinical needs assessment evaluates, answers why one completes a needs assessment, outlines steps when completing the assessment, and discusses processes and key points for obtaining IRB approval. Examples of methods used when completing a needs assessment will be provided. Others may modify or adapt the examples based upon situations, organizational idiosyncrasies, and community needs. A sample of IRB submission criteria is also provided. For purposes of this chapter, two definitions of a needs assessment are provided. First, the World Health Organization (WHO, 2000) defined a needs assessment as a tool for project and program planning. Secondly, a needs assessment is defined as a systematic review of the way things are and the way they should be (Rouda & Kusy, 1995).

While there is no standardized format for a clinical needs assessment, in 2000 WHO identified the following three evaluation components that should be considered and/or adopted in the process.

1. Capacity of services in relation to prevalence and incidence of a syndrome or disease in a specific area
2. The mix of services required and/or desired for a syndrome or disease
3. The coordination of services in a healthcare delivery system whereby entry, transition, and follow-up occurs and is standard practice

Answering why a clinical needs assessment is needed can assist individuals and organizations in several ways, which include the following.

- It allows for prioritizing needs for different community and service populations.
- It assists in making decisions related to the range of services in a specific area or for a certain population.
- It provides answers to the best approach to offer and to balance identified services.

Whatever the case, the goals for completing a clinical needs assessment should be clearly identified, and data collected should build the business case for project funding. Business cases are guided by data that validate inefficiencies, the unpredictable nature in organizations, occupational differences, and interdependencies within systems. The assessment data can also serve as a guide for allocation of funding among several areas by the funding source.

As previously stated, there is no standardized or single purpose format for completing a clinical needs assessment. This can be advantageous to organizations due to differing goals, purposes, and missions. DeWit and Rush (1996) proposed the following four questions to consider when completing the needs assessment. They are:

1. How many or what populations need and will seek services?
2. Is there a need for services across several areas?
3. What are the types of services needed and the capacity to meet the identified needs?
4. Can existing services be coordinated to meet the needs or what is required to improve services?

Several methods or tools can be used to answer these questions. The World Health Organization (2000) offered three different approaches to answer question No. 1 (How many or what populations need and will seek services?): (1) a mortality-based prevalence model, (2) a general population survey, and (3) capture-recapture methods.

Mortality-based prevalence models are user friendly and can be calculated as illustrated in the following example. The total number of individuals with a disorder in a region (A) equals the proportion of individuals who die from the disorder (P). More specifically, the P can be further described to include the total number of deaths from the disorder in a given year in a region (D) divided by the annual death rate from the disorder per 10,000 persons (K).

$$A = P(D/K)$$

A general population survey can be completed by contacting individuals with a random or representative sample and asking questions about a disorder, related symptoms and problems, and perceived need for care. The survey may be accomplished by face-to-face interviews or telephone interviews. As with any survey method, advantages and disadvantages need to be considered, including estimates of the need, difficulty in reaching or contacting individuals, bias, and expenses associated with the survey.

The capture-recapture model requires access to records that are computerized and having statistical expertise available. The advantage of this model is that the sample is tagged initially, and then a proportion of the initial sample is recaptured on the second access of records. This method requires capturing initial data about a disorder or population with subsequent data being recaptured by identifying specific locations or regions where specific needs may persist.

When seeking to answer question No. 2 (Is there a service need across several areas?), a useful method is to compare the need of those seeking treatment with information on problems associated with the disorder and their prevalence. This can assist organizations in determining the type and amount of services that can be offered (WHO, 2000).

Question No. 3 (What are the types of services needed and the capacity to meet the identified needs?) is answered using a client-centered **community needs assessment** (WHO, 2000). This prospective data approach assesses perceptions of service need and complemented by the following:

- Continuum of care assessment (population has varied needs that require different approaches such as care management, early and brief intervention, and/or comprehensive assessment)
- Normative assessment (demand-based need and prior performance outcomes; a highly complex approach that accounts for local variation and is best suited for those with statistical applications)
- Prescriptive models (specify the level of services that will be provided)

Answering question No. 4 (Can existing services be coordinated to meet the needs or what is required to improve services?) is probably the most challenging. Specific measures of service coordination are not as developed as other approaches in terms of reliability and validity (WHO, 2000). Individual biases and the data collection methods and analysis being used when collapsing qualitative data must therefore be considered.

Another approach when an organization is considering the completion of a needs assessment is posed by Rohm and Halback (2010). Their method is the balanced scorecard. Six components are proposed for inclusion in the scorecard, and data can be used beyond the needs assessment process as an organization frames projects and programs and for efficacy. The components are:

1. Assessment
2. Strategy
3. Strategic objectives
4. Strategy mapping
5. Performance measures
6. Strategic initiatives

For organizations that are planning a service project, an assessment of the community's strengths and weaknesses is recommended. As community challenges and assets are learned, opportunities for building projects increased and duplication of services is diminished. Rotary International (2010) identified eight community assessment tools that support the process and benefit effective projects. Each assessment tool and descriptions of each are provided.

The first assessment tool is a survey. In developing the survey, the purpose must be explicitly identified. It will shape questions that will be asked and determine who should be surveyed (the sample). The survey delivery method (computerized, pencil/paper, face-to-face) must be considered, and often the method is tested with a small group before administering.

An asset inventory is the second tool. This may be accomplished by observations conducted by team members in a community and focus on asset identification and their **value** as identified by occupants.

The third tool is community mapping, which indicates different people's perspectives about a community. A map of certain points of interest is developed, and the frequency of visits or use is mapped.

Finding out about work habits of community occupants based on age and gender is accomplished by a daily activities schedule. This tool can help identify whether vocational tools may be useful to improve an area's work efficiency.

The fifth tool is a seasonal calendar. This action identifies changes in labor supply and demand, income fluctuations, food demand and consumption, and demands on public services. Information gleaned helps a community know the best times to consider offering programs or starting projects.

The sixth tool, the community café, is an opportunity tool directed at creating an environment whereby individuals discuss issues and seek answers to frequent questions. Information guides decisions for community agencies on what projects and/or services can be offered in a specific location.

The focus group is the seventh tool that may be used during a community assessment. Focus groups are used to determine preferences and opinions on issues and ideas. The data can be used to decide how best to address issues and incorporate ideas in improvement opportunities.

The final tool is a panel discussion. Experts in a particular field respond to specific questions posed by a facilitator. This can be a significant tool that increases awareness about a topic and becoming more knowledgeable about future opportunities for a community.

The possibility of uncovering potential problems in an organization at the micro, meso, and/or macro level may occur when one is completing a needs assessment as noted in the previous text. Loo (2003) proposed two methods that organizations may consider when problems or issues are identified. The two methods include an issues analysis chart and an issues impact assessment. An issues analysis chart assists in describing the problem, its impact, and required actions. An issues impact assessment is complemented by the former by identifying how the problem(s) may become a barrier to initiating the project and/or the negative impacts if the problems occur as the project is being completed.

Oliva and Rockart (1997) suggested three other considerations when an organization completes a clinical needs assessment: (1) interprogram complementarities, (2) interprogram competition, and (3) interactions among and between programs and services. Whether a project or program was successfully implemented and sustained or not, organizations must assess how previous projects and programs were beneficial to the current endeavor. It should be noted if tools can be used again or modified, and if mind-set changes are a result of changes or complemented by previous activities. Organizations should also assess the benefits or challenges associated with interprogram competition. Efforts can become fragmented and employee motivation can erode, resulting in cynicism and deterioration of management's reputation. Finally, organizations must consider the interactions between programs and services when one program or service is recognized and the contributions of others are underestimated as contributing to the overall successes. **Exhibit 6-1** provides an example of a needs assessment that can be used to provide students guidelines for identifying major concepts and issues in completing this foundational step in project planning. This assignment also provides a case report, further underscoring the need to pursue this project.

Exhibit 6-1

Needs Assessment/Case Report: 20%/100% Course Grade

This exhibit involves an assignment that will provide the background for problem identification considering the need to undertake your particular project. Using a project management methodology, consider problem(s) that need to be addressed in your practice area. Carl Juran (quality improvement guru) describes a project as a problem scheduled for a solution(s). Defining the problem and the need to seek solutions provides a critical component of project planning.

Using a project planning methodology, Lewis (2005) delineates closed-ended and open-ended problems. Closed-ended problems tend to have single solutions; open-ended problems have multiple solutions. Lewis, in support of the importance of constructing a good problem statement, promotes the inclusion of the following items: (1) a clear reflection of shared values and a clear purpose; (2) omitting causes or remedies in the statement itself; (3) defining the problem as manageable processes; (4) including measurable characteristics; and (5) refining statements as evidence (knowledge) is gained.

Consider your needs assessment as you initially define and refine your problem (burning issue). What, as precisely as it can be stated, is the problem? Why is it a problem? For whom is it a problem? Be as concise and clear as possible. Before one can outline project strategies, a clear concise problem statement (based on needs) will be necessary. Examples from your patient population and system will serve as the case report component of this assignment.

Potential alternative solutions need to be outlined as well to form the basis for your project. Your project will address one or potentially more than one of the alternatives detailed in your problem statement as it relates to strategies. You need to consider the pros and cons of each alternative and consider how your selected alternative (your potential project strategies) will address the need.

The six aims for quality improvement can provide a framework for determining need(s). The Institute of Medicine (IOM) describes these aims as follows:

1. Safety: Avoiding injuries to patients from the care that is intended to help them.
2. Effectiveness: Evidence-based services that could help by avoiding overuse and underuse.
3. Patient-centeredness: Respectful care that is responsive to patient values and preferences.

4. Timeliness: Eliminating possible harmful delays for both those who receive and those who provide care.
5. Efficiency: Avoiding waste.
6. Equity: Consistent (does not vary) quality care that is not dependent on gender, ethnicity, geographic location, and socioeconomic status.

Since your project will be focused on quality improvement, you may also consider the 5P Wall model as presented by Baltaden et al. A clear description of the model may be located at http://dms.dartmouth.edu/cms/materials/worksheets.

Using a systems approach to determine need and problem identification can also be useful in describing the background. Tools that may be helpful to this process include those found at the following URLs:

http://www.ceismc.gatech.edu/MM_Tools/analysis.html

http://extension.unh.edu/CommDev/ToolBox/CNATools.ppt#391,2,

Grading Rubric: 20%/100% Course Grade

5 points: Comprehensively describes the need for the project and how need was determined based on the use of a variety of tools (not limited to texts for this course). How is/are your identified need(s) strategically aligned with your system's mission and overall goals?

2 points: Clearly delineates the basic problem; states a concise, comprehensive problem statement, based on a needs assessment. Makes the case for your project within your practice. This is the *so what?* Considers whether the project need is worthy of the costs, resources, stakeholder buy-in, and work involved.

5 points: Effectively summarizes a needs assessment, problem identification, and refined problem statement. The summary includes alternatives/strategies that may address the need/problem. It summarizes the entire assessment in one to two comprehensive yet concise paragraphs and describes the hardcore data (quantitative, qualitative) supporting the need to do this work.

5 points: Identifies and describes a case representative of the problem (concern, issue) and the need to take on this project. This may relate to a particular patient(s) who is the face for your project. Your aggregate data are required in your needs assessment. The case report is a single example of the need,

(continues)

Exhibit 6-1 *(continued)*

serving as an example of how the care (system) would improve if the need is addressed.

3 points: Integrates correct APA style and grammar. Evidences scholarly writing; cites appropriate and timely references liberally throughout the thread and includes a comprehensive reference list. Constructs paragraphs in such a way that they flow from one to another.

20 total possible points.

Source: Institute of Medicine. (2001). *Improving the quality of long-term care.* Washington, DC: National Academy Press.

Once the assessment data are collected and analyzed and plans are developed and implemented, organizations may decide to disseminate information using public forums, conferences, and publications. Organizations must consider human subjects protection and whether information gleaned from assessments can be generalized to the public. Therefore, IRB approval should be secured prior to any data collection.

An institutional review board is a committee mandated by the National Research Act, Public Law 93-348. This law requires that a board be established in a university or other institution that conducts biomedical or behavioral research that involves human subjects. The purpose of the IRB is to review all human subject research proposals, prior to implementation, to assure that the rights of all human rights are protected for those involved in the research. The IRBs emerged based on principles included in the Nuremberg Code, the Declaration of Helsinki, and the Belmont Report. These documents define the minimum codes for conducting research with human beings, as well as beneficence, respect, and justice. Beneficence is addressed by the assessment of risks and benefits to the person; respect is addressed in the informed consent process; and justice is addressed in the process of subject selection.

The IRB is enough to strike fear in the hearts of brave men, but the process is relatively straightforward and procedurally oriented. When one considers the overall purpose, which is to protect human beings, one realizes the process is fairly benign.

Why discuss IRB when quality improvement processes and quality assessments are the foci? If the IRB is predominantly focused on the ethical conduct of research, then why should quality improvement projects be reviewed by the IRB? After all, quality improvement is not research. Patients are the focus of quality improvement/process improvement projects, and their rights must be protected (Speers, 2008). Similarly, community needs assessments can impact individuals and populations; thus protection is warranted.

A notable event in 2007 brought national attention to the impact of quality improvement on patient care and embroiled many professionals in heated arguments about the differences between research and quality improvement. The incident occurred when a major care provider instituted a checklist to remind providers to wash their hands and don sterile gloves and a gown prior to inserting large intravenous lines into patients. Within 3 months of the checklist implementation, infection rates associated with those lines fell precipitously, and the costs associated with them decreased significantly. However, because the checklist was determined to be an intervention that impacted patients and no consent had been obtained from those patients, the Office of Human Research Protection closed down the program. This was done despite the benign nature of the intervention and the significant outcomes realized for patients.

Research is the "systematic investigation . . . designed to develop or contribute to generalizable knowledge" (Speers 2008, p. 1). The intent to publish findings is generally considered as contributing to generalizable knowledge. Quality improvement activities are widely regarded as critical to the effect to reduce healthcare errors and improve patient outcomes, and most can be readily distinguished from research; however, some cannot (Speers, 2008). The issue for students in nurse executive, clinical nurse leader, and doctor of nursing practice programs is that they are not generating new knowledge; instead, they are testing and offering translation of research findings into practice and the care of patients. In order to share with colleagues a project's success in improving quality of care, results are published, which brings quality improvement projects into the realm of research.

As a result of these events, more attention is being paid to process and quality improvement projects and drives the review of projects by IRBs. The problem that most students and project managers face with regard to completion of the application is that the application uses research language, not quality improvement language. Students frequently attempt, in error, to reconcile quality improvement projects with research language, such as describing an experimental design when presenting an intervention. IRB reviewers look for clear explanations of what will be done, who will do it, when it will be done, and how it will be done so that the reviewers can determine if the project requires full board review or is eligible for expedited or exempt status. A clear understanding of the intent of the project is critical to the IRB review process. The list that follows provides some ways to respond to the nature of the question without categorizing the quality improvement project in research terms while assuring ready understanding by IRB review teams. Some of the areas of the application are readily discernable and others take a bit more information.

IRB Submission Criteria

Research purpose. Typically the respondent needs to provide a brief description of the intent of the project for completion.

Subject population. Who will be involved in the project and how?

Design of the study. Address the typical quality improvement designs such as the FADE model (focus, analyze, develop, and execute); PDSA (plan, do, study, act); or Six Sigma (two different models: DMAIC (define, measure, analyze, improve, control) and DMADV (define, measure, analyze, design, verify), which are used for existing or new processes, respectively.

Privacy/confidentiality. How will one protect the information collected? Will participants be recognizable, will responses be linked to participants, etc.? This issue is particularly relevant to staff and/or patients who may fear retribution if they are participants who answer questions truthfully.

Inclusion/exclusion criteria. How will one determine who will participate and who will not? One may not need to use language that is as specific as research language, but one will need to assure that the issue of vulnerability is addressed. If the project does not focus on children, for example, inclusion criteria would reflect over age 19, etc.

Risks/benefits to participate. Even if they are minimal, one needs to address all risks and benefits to the participant, actual or potential, including physical and psychologic risks and benefits, inconvenience, or loss of privacy.

Outcomes. Describe how the information collected will be used. Will the project potentially change practice? How may that change occur? Who will the change affect?

Regardless of the project that is identified, the initial step is to complete a needs assessment, analyze the data, and assimilate data as background support when building the business case. However, one cannot dismiss the need to obtain IRB approval if the data or outcomes of a project will be disseminated beyond the immediate organization or system. Securing IRB approval initially limits future issues.

Summary

- Needs are the cornerstone for project planning.
- Clinical needs and community assessments provide the rationale and support for the project's business case.
- A series of steps is included when completing a clinical needs assessment and a community needs assessment.
- A variety of tools can assist one when completing a needs assessment.
- Institutional review board approval is required for projects where the data will be disseminated beyond the organization. Approval is suggested for internal system data dissemination in support of human subjects' protection.

Reflection Questions

1. What elements are attributed to successful clinical needs assessments and community assessments?
2. What should be considered before beginning the IRB approval process?

References

DeWitt, D. J., & Rush, B. R. (1996). *Evaluation program plan*. Retrieved from http://www.springerlink.com/index/UN5V64N5554LO48W8

Lewis, J. (2005). *Project planning, scheduling, and control*. New York: McGraw-Hill.

Loo, R. (2003). Project management. A core competency for professional nurses and nurse managers. *Journal of Nurses in Staff Development, 19*(4), 187–193.

Oliva, R., & Rockart, S. (1997). *Dynamics of multiple improvement efforts: The program life cycle model*. Retrieved from http://www.systemdynamics.org/conferences/1997/paper166.htm

Rohm, H., & Halbach, L. (2010). A balancing act: Sustaining new directions. *Perform, 3*(2), 1–8.

Rotary International. (2010). *Community assessment tools*. Retrieved from http://www.rotary.rog/newsroom/downloadcenter-pdf5/605c.en.pdf

Rouda, R. H., & Kusy, M. E. (1995). *Needs assessment: The first step*. Retrieved from http://alumnus.caltech.edu/-rouda/T2_NA.html

Speers, M. A. (2008, Spring). Editorial: Quality improvement: Research or non-research? AAHRPP perspective. *Association for the Accreditation of Human Research Protection Programs, Advance, 5*(2), 1–2.

World Health Organization. (2000). *Needs assessment: Workbook 3*. Retrieved from http://www.unodc.org/doc/treatment

SEVEN

Implementing a Project

■ Murielle S. Beene

■ Learning Objectives

1. Identify the steps necessary to implement a project.
2. Discuss midlines as the web of information necessary to be communicated and integrated into the system.
3. Identify leverage and capacity and their relationship to maximizing program efficacy.

> "Plans are only good intentions unless they immediately degenerate into hard work."
>
> —Peter Drucker

Key Terms

Agility
Evidence

Metrics

Roles

Communicator
Decision maker
Implementation project manager
Information manager

Integrator
Leader
Risk anticipator

Professional Values

Altruism
Integrity

Social justice

Core Competencies

Appreciative inquiry
Assessment
Coordination
Critical thinking
Design

Interpersonal influence
Leadership
Management
Risk reduction
Systems thinking

Introduction

Implementation refers to the final process of moving the solution from development status to production status—in other words, where all the planned activities are put into action. The importance of the implementation phase and its significance to project success cannot be understated. The role of the implementation project manager is essential to this accomplishment. This individual possesses characteristics of strong communication skills, is results oriented, understands organization, and is committed to corporate values. There is a close and mutually reinforcing (supportive) relationship between planning, implementation, and monitoring. This chapter discusses the value of collaboration in project implementation and the role of the implementation project manager. A description of a systems change model is provided as an example that can assist readers to answer key questions that support project implementation and sustainability practice settings.

Planning for Implementation

A successful implementation begins with the creation of an executable work plan. The implementation project manager is responsible for crafting the details of this plan, which includes defining goals, objectives, and strategies; developing a timeline; establishing project milestones; and matching project tasks with resources. During the planning process, it is also important to consider overall aims, goals, outcomes, costs, and budgets simultaneously.

As discussed in Chapter 5, the project manager leads the team in conducting a SWOT analysis, identifying strengths and weaknesses (internal forces), opportunities, and threats (external forces). The strengths and opportunities are positive forces that can be expedited to efficiently implement a project. Weaknesses and threats may hamper project implementation, if they are not considered in light of the overall aims and context of the project. Many organizations simultaneously conduct a needs assessment and a SWOT analysis and then compare findings. The needs assessment focuses on a summary of the following areas:

- Descriptions of the qualitative and quantitative data that support the need for the project.
- The costs, resources, stakeholder buy-in, and work requirements necessary for a successful and meaningful project outcome prior to implementation.
- Determination of whether need(s) are strategically aligned with the organization's mission and overall goals.

The information gleaned from the needs assessment is pivotal and requires comprehensive considerations prior to planning and implementing a project. The role of the implementation project manager transitions into risk anticipator, assisting project stakeholders in devising a strategy means of overcoming potential barriers. It is best to begin with the end in mind. That is, what is the expectation for quality outcomes when undertaking a project initiative? Lighter (2011) identified the need for stakeholders to consider the value proposition when implementing a project. More specifically, he proposed the following formula to calculate value:

$$Value = quality/cost$$

Inherent in the planning process is the development of an implementation strategy. The implementation strategy is meant to focus on the process from a stakeholder perspective and should be approved prior to execution. The most common implementation strategy is the phased approach for a project (Glaser, 2009). This approach is relatively safe for the organization because it allows the project team members to reassess after each project phase is operationalized. For example, in a project to reduce catheter-acquired urinary tract infections (CAUTIs), phases may include determination of the extent of the problem, using data to drive urgency to act (magnitude of problem), outcomes to be measured, implementation strategies, and evaluation protocols.

A key document in the implementation phase is a project charter. A project charter is an agreement between the organization providing the service and the stakeholder requesting the service and receiving the deliverables (Lewis, 2005). The project charter includes a comprehensive description of the project, a list of anticipated project team members, and their specific roles and responsibilities in the project. Also included in the charter is the level of authority for the project manager and the project outcomes. The charter outlines the scope and measures of success with formal signatures for project authorization and approval. This process is critical to building consensus on project goals and documents communication between project stakeholders. For example, a project aimed at reducing catheter-acquired urinary tract infections (CAUTIs) on an acute surgical unit may involve the clinical nurse leader (CNL), infection control nurse, a patient representative, and staff nurses. The CNL may take the lead as project manager, outlining particular roles of each member (observing how patients' urinary catheters are handled during transport, monitoring the number of catheters inserted, discontinued, etc.). Setting up communication channels, meeting times, and review tools may also be established and delegated by the CNL. While other team members are intimately involved in the implementation and have an active voice in all project-related measures, the CNL is the project manager, but cannot and should not be expected to produce the project outcomes alone.

Another phase of the project implementation may include an action plan (based on the best available **evidence**) that delineates particular strategies. The action plan includes the following elements:

- How evidence-based interventions will be used to improve the system (system's change) and practice
- The *what* and *how* to accomplish the stated purpose
- The collaboration and teamwork required to implement the project, its sustainability, and its relevance to an existing program or mission
- Information flow processes (informatics and technology)
- Interventions that will focus on educating others about the project and how the information provided will guide stakeholders throughout the implementation phase and result in the stated project goal/aim
- Descriptions of the theoretical or conceptual underpinnings and their relevance to the overall project and program mission
- How organizational and cultural dynamics will be addressed
- Anticipated impacts that the project will have and how findings close gaps identified by the SWOT analysis and needs assessment
- Time-specific milestones

An evaluation phase to measure success of actions taken is important to determine the efficacy of the plan. An evaluation plan includes the following:

- Methods and **metrics** for evaluating the project
- Timelines and data milestones
- Measurement types that include structure, process, and outcome
- Metrics that evidence relevance to stakeholders and the system, are scientifically sound, and are associated with processes that can be modified through reasonable methods and procedures

Lessons learned, barriers that were overcome during the implementation phase, and strategies used to overcome the barriers could further inform the project.

Micro-, Meso-, and Macrocollaboration

Collaboration across organizational stakeholders requires communication, commitment, accountability, and continuity (McElmurry et al., 2009). In order to ensure that a new initiative is realized to its full potential, stakeholders must see the strategic alignment. Administrative support for a project may enhance successful implementation and sustainability. For example, reducing CAUTIs aimed at reducing patient's discomfort and costs of care serve to advance the mission of the organization, thus addressing the overall mission of quality: safe care. The implementation project manager translates to stakeholders how existing business processes would be improved with project implementation. Project stakeholders (project sponsors, decision makers, and leaders) in a healthcare organization publicly endorsing the project may underscore the importance of the project's purpose.

With the implementation of a project, the significance associated with collaboration with stakeholders is priceless. Therefore, it is important to involve organizational stakeholders from the beginning, provide intermittent progress checks, be responsive to concerns, and address risks throughout implementation. At the point of implementation, the implementation project manager ensures resource needs are clear and project risks are reviewed and validated. Stakeholder expectations must be managed during implementation through continued focus on the strategic goal for the project (McElmurry et al., 2009). Structure, process, and outcome indicators are continually evaluated to assure that resources are being used efficiently and effectively. Meetings to share progress and lessons learned, for example, actual reduction in CAUTIs, further enhance credibility of the project team's work.

Communicate, Communicate, and Communicate

In addition to planning and collaboration, the other fundamental element of implementation is communication. The purpose of communications management is to share the right information, at the right time, with the right people, and in the right format. Good communications management means expending effort on communicating information, which contributes to project success; lack of information can lead to failure. Most importantly, the implementation project manager must identify the correct target audience for different categories of communications.

Strong communication must be accompanied by mutual trust. Both formal and informal methods can be used to disseminate information. Formal communication methods follow well-defined, systematic procedures, while informal communications are casual and more extemporaneous. Weekly status reports containing information about progress and issues are examples of a formal communication tool. Some examples of informal communication include voice mail, e-mail, and text messages. An effective and perhaps an efficient method of conveying information within a team is face-to-face conversation. The implementation plan should be circulated to all stakeholders involved in the project. The implementation project manager communicates continually to reinforce the messages and make sure everyone is ready when implementation occurs. The management of communication is implemented through three essential processes. The processes are:

1. **Identification**: Process of identifying information to be shared, when it should be distributed, who should receive it, and how it should be prepared
2. **Reporting**: Process of collecting and preparing the information
3. **Distribution**: Process of disseminating the information, and for formal communications, storing the information in the project archive

Change Management

Change management is possibly the most important factor in the implementation process. For example, when a healthcare organization is adopting a clinical or financial information system, there are significant changes to its business processes, so there will be a definite learning curve. The change process must be actively managed. Change management may be led by someone external to the organization, possibly a consultant, and begins at the start of implementation. This individual or group of individuals would collaborate with the implementation project manager and project stakeholders to craft a change management blueprint tailored for the organization.

An effective change management technique is to adopt a department to test the new approach. Rather than a big-bang start, it is often more productive to begin with one department; this requires one unit or department to test the project initiative. A staged approach allows the implementation project manager and stakeholders to monitor the initiative at work on a small scale and react to any resulting issues. This steady progression generates confidence and understanding throughout the organization, building buy-in for the project. This gradual process of integration can be replicated with employees as well. They are encouraged to start off slowly and build their knowledge and confidence related to the project initiative.

Faculty members from the University of South Alabama College of Nursing developed a model that visually illustrates the intersecting aspects of a system change project that can assist organizations and students when planning and implementing a project. It is shown in **Figure 7-1**. Questions are posed for each intersecting aspect

Figure 7–1   System change project intersecting aspects.

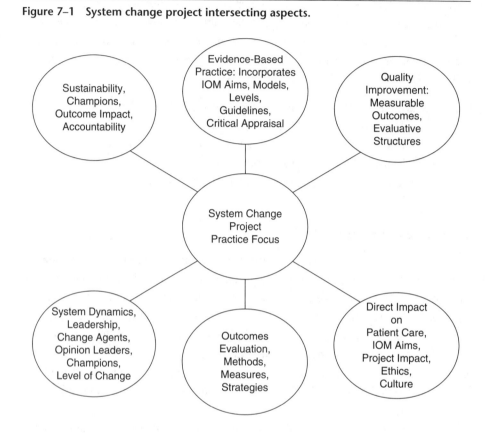

that can guide the implementation of the system change project. The intersecting aspects and accompanying questions are presented:

Evidence-Based Practice: Incorporates IOM Aims, Models, Levels, Guidelines, Critical Appraisal

1. Is there a model or framework of how evidence is managed?
2. Are level(s) identified?
3. Is there a critical appraisal mechanism?

Quality Improvement: Measurable Outcomes, Evaluative Structures

1. Is a model/framework plan in place?
2. What is the quality improvement process?

Direct Impact on Patient Care, IOM Aims, Project Impact, Ethics, Culture

1. Are the aims clearly defined?
2. What is the direct impact on patient care?

Outcomes Evaluation, Methods, Measures, Strategies

1. Are outcomes defined?
2. Are measures to be evaluated identified?
3. Are methods to evaluate outcomes defined?

System Dynamics, Leadership, Change Agents, Opinion Leaders, Champions, Level of Change

1. Is there a conceptual/theoretical framework identified?
2. Is it integrated into the project plan?
3. What system(s) are to be changed?
4. Who are the change agents? Opinion leaders? Change champions?
5. Is this an incremental change? Transformational change? How do you know?

Sustainability, Champions, Outcome Impact, Accountability

1. Do long-term plans exist?
2. What plans are in place to maintain sustainability?

Resistance to Change Is a Reality—Embrace It

Training and education play an important role in overcoming resistance in the adoption of new organizational initiatives. Research revealed that adult learners have the capability to grasp new information early in the implementation phase of a project (Bond, 2006). The implementation project manager must collaborate with educational resources within the organization to develop training materials in the planning process of this project. Equally important is the support of decision makers and leadership in providing these resources to support project efforts.

Postproject Monitoring and Evaluation

Projects should be continuously evaluated for quality and appropriateness. Adjustments can be made at the time of discovery, instead of at the end-of-project implementation (Kitzmiller, Hunt, & Sproat, 2006). In this case, the project may have more minor, smaller adjustments instead of larger, more costly swings in project scope and direction.

Postimplementation reviews can be conducted to identify value achievement progress and the steps still needed to achieve maximum gain. It is extremely rare that healthcare organizations revisit their investments to determine whether promised value was actually achieved (Glaser, 2009). Some organizations believe that once the implementation is over and the change settles in, value will automatically be achieved (Glaser). Healthcare organizations should conduct reviews of projects periodically to evaluate progress.

Postimplementation reviews support the achievement of value by signaling leadership interest in ensuring the delivery of results, identifying the steps to ensure value, and reinforcing accountability for results.

- What goals were expected at the time the project was approved?
- How close have we come to achieving project goals?
- How much has the organization invested into the project, and how does it compare with original budget?
- If we had to implement the project again, what would we do differently?

Monitoring is an important component of the implementation phase in order to ensure that the project is implemented per the schedule. This is a continuous process that should be put in place before project implementation starts. These monitoring activities should be executed by all individuals and institutions that have an interest (stakeholders) in the project. To efficiently implement a project, the people planning and implementing it should plan for all the interrelated stages from the beginning. Metrics are also important to ensure that activities are implemented as planned. This helps the implementation project manager to measure how well he or she is achieving project milestones and goals. As such, the monitoring activities should appear on the work plan and should involve all stakeholders. If project activities are not going well, arrangements should be made to identify the problem so that they can be corrected.

Organizations should benchmark their performance in achieving value against the performance of like organizations (Glaser, 2009). These benchmarks may focus on process performance to use data to inform everything from resource allocation to instructional practice. Stakeholders, especially project sponsors, should understand the accountability they have for the successful completion of the project. There should be an agreed-upon set of metrics that will be used to track value delivery. These metrics should be in addition to the metrics used to evaluate project implementation.

Project Implementation Challenges

There are many potential implementation challenges for a project. Some of the common ones include funding and the management of stakeholders. Due to numerous stakeholders that would be directly involved in the project, there will undoubtedly be some political challenges. Another frequent implementation challenge is the lack of communication among stakeholders, leadership, and the implementation project manager. This miscommunication creates divergence in perception of critical initiatives that have great potential to benefit a healthcare organization.

Some common reasons of project implementation failure are a result of poor communication with leadership and stakeholders, organizational resistance to change, scope creep, lack of project ownership and champion, and/or shifts in organizational priorities. The recommended approach in achieving implementation success is the incorporation of agility concept into the project process (Kitzmiller et al., 2006). Agility is a concept that encourages flexibility, adaptation, and continuous learning as a part of the implementation process. The agility process is an approach that accepts the complexity of a problem and addresses it through frequent inspection, responding with a flexible approach of constant adaption (Kitzmiller et al., 2006). Agility considers the complexity of the problems faced in the current healthcare environment and enhances traditional implementation techniques.

Summary

- Implementation is the final process of moving the solution from development to production status.
- Successful implementation begins with an executable plan.
- A SWOT analysis and needs assessment are critical to successful project implementation.
- Project charters identify outcomes that can be tracked.
- Collaboration requires communication among and between all stakeholders.
- A systems change project considers several aspects that impact practice outcomes.

Reflection Questions

1. Identify two aspects of project planning that will assure success, and compare these to situations in daily practice.
2. Identify factors to consider when dealing in external forces and barriers that can impede project implementation.

Learning Activity

Consider a project that you have implemented and identify strengths, weakness, threats, and opportunities of your approach to implementing the project.

References

Bond, G. E. (2006). Lessons learned from the implementation of web-based nursing intervention. *Computers in Nursing, 24(2),* 66–71.

Glaser, J. (2009). A strategy for ensuring a project delivers value. *Healthcare Financial Management, 63(7),* 28–31.

Kitzmiller, R., Hunt, E., & Sproat, S. (2006). Adopting best practices: Agility moves from software development to healthcare project management. *Computers in Nursing, 24*(2), 75–82.

Lewis, J. (2005). Project planning, scheduling, and control. New York: McGraw-Hill.

Lighter, D. E. (2011). *Advanced performance improvement in health care.* Sudbury, MA: Jones and Bartlett.

McElmurry, B. J., McCreary, L. L., Park, C. G., Ramos, L., Martinez, E., Parikh, R., et al. (2009). Implementation, outcomes, and lessons learned from a collaborative primary health care program to improve diabetes care among urban Latino populations. *Health Promotion Practice, 10*(2), 293–302.

EIGHT

The Role of Information Technology and the Enterprise in Project Planning and Implementation

■ James L. Harris, Murielle S. Beene, Pam Pickett, Mimi Haberfelde, Alicia Levin, and Bonny Collins

■ **Learning Objectives**

1. Identify key stakeholders and leader roles necessary to develop information technology (IT) products that support projects and programs.
2. Discuss the importance of IT for success in an organization.
3. Identify IT enablers common to project development and program success.
4. Discuss the importance of IT skills sets in a global economy.
5. Use IT products for education and program successes.

> "The hardest thing is not to get people to accept new ideas; it is to get them to forget old ones."
>
> —John Maynard Keynes

> "Wisdom consists not so much in knowing what to do in the ultimate, as knowing what to do next."
>
> —Herbert Hoover

Key Terms

Collaboration

Information technology

Information technology enterprise

Project leadership

Project performance

Roles

Collaborator

Communicator

Information manager

Integrator

Project leader

Professional Values

Inquisitiveness

Objectivity

Social justice

Core Competencies

Systems thinking

Design

Management

Risk reduction

Leadership

Communication

Information technology knowledge

Knowledge

Risk anticipation

Systems thinking

Introduction

As introduced in preceding chapters, communication, **project leadership**, synergy, team interactions, planning, and implementation of projects must be considerate of the role of **information technology** (IT) and how the **information technology enterprise** drives decisions and ultimate success. In an era of a technology-driven business decisions, knowing how to use technology and tools in support of projects and for sustainability of projects is key to success. With the myriad of challenges confronting healthcare organizations, projects that are being planned must (1) capitalize on the talents and skills of teams; (2) support and expand program capacity;

(3) capitalize on available IT tools that support projects; and (4) gain operational efficiency (Anantatmula, 2008; Smith, 2001). Despite the advances in IT, it is not uncommon for projects to fail for a variety of reasons, which is further validation of the importance of technology and the IT enterprise (Williams, 2005).

In this chapter, the complexities of healthcare environments are addressed, as are the role of technology and the enterprise for success when planning and implementing projects, lived experiences of nurses who plan projects for national implementation, and their interface with informatics staff. Specific project examples and deliverables that evidence project needs, IT process requirements and activities associated with the project, and valuable tools of the trade are provided.

Stakeholder and Leadership Involvement

Similar to traditional nursing practice, it is recommended that project management practices include the documentation of the scope, milestones, risks, and issues from project initiation to evaluation. Documentation may prove to be invaluable in promoting successful project completion. Project implementation success begins with senior leadership commitment from both nursing and IT. Cleland (1995) identified that a project's success or failure is directly related to the leadership of project stakeholders. Thite (1999) reinforced that leadership is a critical success factor for projects, and the size of a project determines the degree of leadership involvement. Projects that capitalize on IT systems and have leaders who exhibit transformational and technical leadership behaviors are historically successful.

Project stakeholders must participate in all phases of project management to ensure that interests are adequately represented. It is imperative that there is dedicated project sponsorship and leadership to support the initiative. A large body of literature reveals that using a project management approach results in more effective and efficient management in a variety of organizational contexts including health care. Therefore, advocates can convince executive management of the benefits of implementing project management (Anantatmula, 2008).

It is important that the introduction and effectiveness of project management be evaluated, if, in fact, project management improves the effectiveness and efficiency of projects as well as the skills of participating staff in both the technical and nursing side of management. This systematic review demonstrates that project evaluation in healthcare facilities is of significant interest to administrators, nurses, the nursing profession, and to furthering nursing knowledge.

Information Technology Supporting Projects and Programs

Information technology allows healthcare organizations and providers to store and retrieve data quickly while creating an option to meet the dual mandate, which is to achieve excellence in quality and efficiency. Continuous human actions are required to convert information to knowledge. However, Prieto and Revilla (2004) pointed out that humans are slower than IT systems in converting data into information. Therefore, improved communication and bridging the gap between IT and end users will assist in communicating data to others and be useful information that can support project development, implementation, and sustainability in the long term.

As healthcare organizations consider new projects that complement or expand existing programs, IT investment is necessary for improving **project performance** and creating a competitive edge over others, but as Anantatmula (2008) suggested, performance, impact, and outcomes of a project depend on how IT systems are designed and on the relationship to other business and organizational metrics. Successful project and program sustainability is influenced by accumulated knowledge and individual and collective competence (Kasvi, Vartiainen, & Hailikari, 2003). But considering that individuals move within and among organizations, additional project and program duties may be assumed, and project metrics change, the importance of IT systems in reducing variability and redundancy through data capture and storage cannot be overstated (Karlsen & Gottschalk, 2004).

Information Technology as Positive Enabler for Project Planning and Program Management

When one maps processes involved with tasks that ultimately support project and program success, it is not uncommon to discover the number of steps that staff takes to complete a task. For example, when a nurse contacts pharmacy about the status of a medication that was ordered hours before, this can require numerous steps, which costs money and may be better delegated to another staff member. IT systems are proposed as an enabler for resolving such issues, reducing steps and redundancies, consequently improving processes. The California Healthcare Foundation and First

Consulting Group (2002) identified several enablers that positively support many programs and are used by many organizations. The enablers are:

- Mobile communication devices.
- Automated nurse scheduling systems that allow nurses to bid on specific shifts.
- Computerized order entry and patient documentation.
- Secure messaging and e-mail.
- Automated documentation templates.
- Medication administration and management inventory systems.

Turisco and Rhoads (2008) stated that IT systems have the potential to create a better work environment and can have a dramatic impact on organizational operations. Removing staff from tasks and the communication chain that do not require certain skill sets, using technologies to assist in work organization and clinical decision support, using technologies for instruction and education, and integrating wireless technology with monitoring devices enable staff to respond in a timely way and are other examples of how IT can be viewed as an enabler to successful project development and ongoing program management. Another pointed example of how IT is a positive enabler for staff was illustrated in a comment from a new graduate nurse who was working in an organization that is paperless for documentation and a system failure occurred. The employee commented to administrators, "The time it took for handwritten documentation was extreme due to the difficulty writing succinct information and rereading entries to assure correct grammar and completeness."

Building a Skill Set for Nurses Who Develop Projects and Manage Programs: The Information Technology Link

Whether developing an administrative dashboard or clinical application product, IT is required for nurses and nurse leaders to thrive in an information-driven society (Runy, 2008). Not all nurses need to be superusers, but a basic knowledge of IT is needed. Leaders cannot delegate this skill requirement to others. In today's environment, IT becomes a thread woven throughout the organization. Nurses and leaders, armed with knowledge, build the business case (the argument) and the business plan (the document) for structuring IT initiatives, goals for implementation and metrics, and accountability for implementation. The escalating drum beat for operational efficiency requires nurses and other healthcare team members to data mine (discover knowledge) large data sets in order to design and/or redesign new models of care delivery and efficiency models. These activities inevitably require IT skill sets, both general and advanced.

The need for healthcare organizations to be skilled users and consumers of IT is underscored by the partnership of educators and administrators to develop skills of end users. Nursing has made great progress in educating nurses about IT and the enterprise by incorporating content into basic and advanced degree-granting programs. As these skills are developed, nurses are using technologic advances to communicate with patients, families, and other team members remotely. Health information is growing exponentially. E-nursing, the use of existing data and information and communication technology, is revolutionizing the way nurses interact with patients and teams and learn new or enhanced skill sets. In today's era of IT and home technology, multiple interactive media are available to educate patients and families, and through simulation, staff has opportunities to master skills necessary for quality and safe care. Nurses are also being educated using blend learning (on-site and online), thus enhancing skills and abilities to meet the demands of the healthcare consumer. IT has multiple advantages and will expand only as providers are prepared to meet the healthcare needs of citizens globally.

Clinical and Administrative Information Technology Product Examples and Processes

The following text discusses the experiences of nurses who have developed IT projects for a federally funded healthcare organization.

Product Focus: Nurse-Sensitive Indicators Development

In 2002, the Veterans Health Administration (VHA) Office of Nursing Services (ONS) initiated the Veterans Administration (VA) Nursing Outcomes Database (VANOD) project with the intent of developing a national database of clinically relevant acute care nursing indicators. The project was modeled after the California Nursing Outcomes Coalition project, the largest statewide nursing quality indicators project in the nation. According to the VANOD manual, the overall goal of the initiative was to assure VA administrators, nurse executives, and quality managers that nurse staffing in VA settings was positively related to patient care outcomes. A VHA nursing outcomes database of quality indicators would ultimately improve care to veterans because valid, reliable, and quantitative data will enable ongoing examination of processes and relationships between nurse-sensitive patient outcomes and structural/ organizational elements. For example, after risk adjustment, analyses would depict the relationship between staffing variables and pressure ulcers or between staffing variables and patient falls. The database would enable testing of practices, provide an evidence base for assessment and interventions, and determine relationships between the structure and processes of nursing care. The database was being designed to generate reports that can be used for comparative purposes and for research studies related to structure, process, and outcomes across the VHA.

A 16-month pilot project was initiated with 12 pilot facilities manually collecting data and submitting it to the project coordinators for analysis and reporting. Initial indicators included:

- Nursing hours per patient day
- Skill mix
- Patient falls
- Pressure ulcer prevalence
- Nursing staff musculoskeletal patient-handling injuries
- Patient satisfaction
- RN satisfaction

The process of manually collecting and submitting data indicated the need for a standardized, automated approach for data collection and reporting. Manual reporting was replaced with the extraction of administrative data from existing files—paid files and the human resource files available within the system. The electronic data extraction and reporting was the result of **collaboration** among all stakeholders, including VANOD staff, programmers, nurse executives, and VANOD and Magnet coordinators. Continued cycles of refinement resulted in the deployment of national skin-care assessment templates and resulting reports.

Cycles of Refinement for VANOD Nursing Indicators

The following information outlines the cycles of refinement associated with VANOD nursing indicators.

- Manual data gathered at pilot facilities
- Reports analyzed and provided to pilot facilities
- Electronic data extraction developed
- Reports created from human resources files and paid files available at the national, network, and local levels
- Annual RN satisfaction survey conducted
- Results available at the national, network, and local levels
- Skin-care clinical documentation template deployed nationally
- Clinical indicator data available at the national, network, and facility level to the treating specialty
- Granularity to nurse location (unit level) in process

Each cycle of refinement represents collaboration with partners and a systematic process of planning deployment to include testing of the product(s), end user education, and initial and ongoing validation of data. Products have been developed for staff in various roles (i.e., the nurse executive dashboard and the VANOD annual summary report) based upon input solicited from end users. Ongoing educational programs, frequent conference calls with stakeholders, and the deployment of comprehensive data definition documents were key to the initial and ongoing success of this program. Throughout the evolution of these products and reports, ongoing collaboration between VANOD project leaders and stakeholders was and remains essential to its success.

Sample Report Access Format

Data may be reviewed in various formats that include the following:

- **ProClarity cubes**: Allows for robust customization of data views.
- **Briefing Books**: Presents users with preestablished reports that allow for limited customization and drill-down of data.

- **MS Reporting Services format**: A report that allows users to view national, network, and local level data with limited customization. All formats allow users to export data to various applications for further analysis. Links to data definitions and supporting documentation are available to users within each reporting application.

Reference

VA Nursing Outcomes Database Program Manual (Acute Care version). (2005, Sept.). Retrieved from http://vaww.collage.research.med.va.gov/collage/VANOD/new/ workbook.asp

Product Focus: Skin Risk

Business Reason for Project

Pressure ulcer prevention is an important patient safety goal. According to the Institute for Healthcare Improvement, 1 million people develop pressure ulcers annually, while approximately 60,000 acute care patients die from related complications. Pressure ulcer prevalence has been recognized as a nursing-sensitive indicator in nursing databases, including the National Database for Nursing Quality Indicators and the California Nursing Outcomes Coalition. In 2009, Medicare began to deny payment for preventable hospital-acquired conditions, which include stage III and IV pressure ulcers.

National pressure ulcer prevention and incidence information has been lacking across the VA system because of lack of consistent data source and lack of methodology for data capture. In early 2007, VANOD began reviewing a sample of skin risk indicators through chart review for specific patient cohorts, until an automated documentation system could be developed and implemented. In October 2007, two nationally standardized skin risk nursing documentation templates were released to the facilities, providing the ability to document skin inspection and pressure ulcer risk on admission as well as periodic reassessment during the patient's hospital stay. Both of these templates were mandated for acute care settings, with relevant data elements tagged for capture during the process of documentation.

The intended purpose of providing the VANOD skin risk data is to:

- Detail information about skin risk nursing processes and patient outcomes.
- Determine care burden related to pressure ulcer cases.
- Improve patient safety.
- Increase service quality to veterans.

The Stakeholders

Stakeholders include all VA administrative and clinical staff within the central office, VA regional offices, and at the medical center or facility level. There are two large enterprise-wide e-mail distribution lists of wound ostomy continence care nurses, for whom this information is important, as a way of determining improvements in nursing processes and patient care outcomes.

Implementation Strategy

Template Development

Using the VA *Pressure Ulcer Prevention Handbook* and The Joint Commission as supporting evidence, skin risk nursing process and patient outcomes indicators were identified. Initial development of the documentation tool was completed using nine wound-care nurses from across the system and a programmer from the Office of Health Information. During a series of conference calls, content was created and refined to be consistent with the VHA *Pressure Ulcer Prevention Handbook* as well as The Joint Commission and national patient safety goals. Following development of relevant, desired indicators, data elements were tagged within the templates to enable later data capture.

The participating wound care nurses' facilities were used as the testing ground for initial use of the pilot template. Each site had five nurses use the template based on supplied patient care scenarios or actual local examples. Feedback was provided for change recommendations. Following changes, the new template was retested, and the templates submitted to the Office of Information and Technology for final testing and deployment to the facilities.

Prerelease Data Validation

Three months prior to national implementation, 11 volunteer pilot sites were invited to participate in a 6-week process to test a data validation process of extracted skin risk data. Additional one-on-one calls occurred with individual sites during this time frame for troubleshooting purposes.

Sites were provided with instructions for obtaining patient-level data access, and a Web link tool was created with the following features:

- Numbers and calculated scores for each of the indicators by month from January through April
- Data by admitting specialty for patients discharged during that month (all patients were admitted after January)
- Patient data at the Social Security Number level (for authorized users) so that individual chart review was possible
- Links to the following:
  o A skin risk data definitions document (indicator statements and calculations)
  o A data validation tool (Excel spreadsheet for indicator validation documentation)
  o Ad hoc report instructions for reviewing individual patient data within the computerized patient record system

Validation was completed by only 45% of the group, but findings were consistent. Data quality issues seemed to be in regard to the facility data transmission to the national database. Observation and preadmitted patients were not being captured. Prevalence studies, if completed during the month prior to patient discharge, had some usefulness as a comparator. The ability to look at individual patient charts, as well as to run a specialized report to view if the data elements were being captured, was helpful. Local nursing documentation variance and educational needs were identified, including:

- Use of the incorrect template (i.e., reassessment rather than initial on admission)
- Incorrect pressure ulcer staging, misidentification of pressure ulcers, and no documentation of existing pressure ulcers were all identified as additional areas of educational needs.

One of the pilot sites created and shared a methodology for running a report on local identified patients to determine if their data elements were tagged in a way that indicated use of the correct template. This methodology has proven to be of great benefit to the system in the data validation process.

Template Release

The templates were released nationally by the Office of Information and Technology with installation instructions. Advance notice was provided to sites, with announcements on all relevant calls. Educational tools and information were posted to the VANOD website, including a facility PowerPoint slide show with screen prints and relevant information about the template, including what to use when and a frequently asked questions document. Weekly national calls occurred during the release month, and the calls included VANOD staff, programmers, and representatives from Office of Information and Technology for open questions and answers.

Communication

During the process of indicator and template development, intent and project status was announced on standing conference calls with leadership and the field through the monthly VANOD nurse executive calls, field advisory council, and VANOD site coordinator calls. The project website (VANOD website) was used to post educational tools, including a PowerPoint slide show with screen prints of the template and information on its use. The quarterly VANOD newsletter has wide distribution across the system, and articles were included regarding initiation, status, and release of the templates.

Product Examples

Reports are housed on a national database, accessible to anyone within the VA. Patient -level or protected access data cannot be viewed unless the proper security permissions are applied for and granted. Reports are created in three formats that are useful to the casual user or more advanced user. The more advanced format is flexible and dynamic with existing reports that can be sliced and diced according to the viewer's data need.

Product examples include the following:

- Skin risk assessment within 24 hours of admission, including ability to drill to facility level or by month and medical specialty
- National, network, or facility indicator summary report, including ability to view indicator summary report by month and from VHA down to network or facility level
- Patient outcomes-hospital-acquired pressure ulcer rate

Evaluation

Since initial templates release to present:

- Rate of patients assessed within 24 hours of admission rose from 51% to 85%.
- Rate of patients with documentation of daily skin inspection rose from 14% to 41%.
- Trends for assessment and pressure ulcer documentation are beginning to more closely align with comparative data.

A national view of VA skin care nursing processes and patient care outcomes is now available and has provided impetus for change. Issues identified included problems with the template fitting into the nursing work flow and educational needs in relation to pressure ulcer identification. Challenges and successes with skin risk have paved the way for development of a user-friendly, comprehensive patient documentation package, which will enable capture of additional key nursing-sensitive indicators.

Project Focus: RN Satisfaction

Business Reason for Project

Improving nurse satisfaction is key to recruitment and especially to retention of registered nurses (RNs) and is thus of high importance to the VA. Annual surveys of registered nurses' satisfaction with the structural and qualitative aspects of their work environment, for the purposes of analysis and improvement, are therefore critical. At a national level, annual surveys provide a trended view of RN satisfaction across the system, while at the facility level, analysis of RN satisfaction results provides an action planning tool to maintain positive findings and/or improve negative findings.

Based on initial pilot work in 2004–2005, it was obvious that to provide a survey across a system as large as VA, Web-based access to the survey and to reports was critical to rapid, easy survey access and submission, as well as reporting. Therefore in 2006, the first national VA RN satisfaction survey was deployed via a link from the VA Nursing Outcomes Database (VANOD) website. Resulting data from the reports were housed in the VANOD database in a flexible format that provided basic reports with the ability for stakeholders to slice and dice the data in a variety of ways for improved analysis. The survey now occurs on an annual basis and now also includes trend reports for the last 4 years of data.

The Stakeholders

The RN satisfaction survey process and reports database was developed by VANOD in collaboration with the Veterans Integrated Services Network (VISN) Support Service Center (VSSC); Healthcare Talent Management Office, the National Center for Organizational Development; and the Health Services Research & Development (HSR&D) Center for Organizational Leadership, Management and Research in Boston, Massachusetts, which are also all key stakeholders in the annual national all-employee survey. This collaborative approach provides the resources needed for field support; survey programming and data management; results analysis using correlation and statistical significance; and customizable reports for national, regional, and field use. This collaboration is also important in assisting VHA facilities to analyze the results, while maintaining anonymity for survey respondents. Other stakeholders include administrative and clinical staff within the central office, VHA regional offices, and at the medical center or facility level.

At the facility level, RN satisfaction data provides information to nursing stakeholders for the development of RN recruitment and retention planning. The six topic scales (participation, quality of care, staffing, nurse manager, RN/MD relations, and IT support) provide a global topic score, with the ability to hone in on specific questions. Identified high scores can be supported, while lower scores provide a focus for improvement. The ability to trend over time provides facilities the opportunity to compare against their own performance year to year, as well as to the VHA average and best scoring VA as their benchmarks. Facility results can be shared among managers and staff to provide a way of thinking about what they can do to strengthen their organization. Survey results provide the ONS workforce development team with data for improvement opportunities and support across the system.

Implementation Strategy

The implementation strategy consists of the following activities:

Presurvey Implementation

Leadership Communication. Management and medical center leadership briefings begin 6 months prior to survey kickoff. Venues include regular VA medical center management conference calls as a way of introducing the purpose, plan, and process for the RN satisfaction survey. The monthly ONS national nurse executive and nurse manager calls provide a venue for questions and answers. Additional tools include articles in the quarterly Office of Nursing Services Informatics (ONSI) newsletter, including background and plan; messages posted on the VANOD website; and team contact information posted in both places.

Site Communication and Tools. Monthly conference calls with designated facility site coordinators begin 6 months prior to the survey. Volunteers are requested to participate in a 6-week process to develop and evaluate a survey marketing tool, providing their wisdom on what worked well at their facility or what they wish they had done differently in prior surveys. A marketing tool is created, including a survey road map and customizable posters, letters, and staff instructions in accessing the survey for use at the facility level. Weekly e-mails to the site coordinators are sent by the survey team during the final month prior to survey kickoff.

Postimplementation

- Motivational e-mails on the day of survey kickoff.
- An RN response rate link from the ONS VANOD website, enabling sites to see facility progress in real time.
- Weekly motivational e-mails to facility leadership and site coordinators.
- Contact phone numbers for survey technical assistance (within the survey itself) or to contact the survey team (on the survey website) are provided so that concerns or issues can rectified and logged.

Postsurvey. Once the survey has closed (at midnight Pacific time on October 31st), the survey administration team begins the process of data validation checks prior to sending to the research and reports teams. Further data validation is done between the corresponding software packages to ensure that counts are matching, prior to development of the national and facility survey analysis and reports creation.

The Veterans Integrated Services Network (VISN) Support Service Center houses the data set within the VANOD database and collaborates with the VANOD team on report format. Once the data validation, data analysis, and reports creation are completed, data are posted, usually by mid-January. Data results at the VHA level are shared in the regular executive level meetings and with the site coordinators. An e-mail is sent to executive level management including facility directors and nurse executives, as well as to site coordinators, with a link to the reports. Educational PowerPoint slide shows are posted on the VANOD website and presented at relevant conference calls. Typical nursing questions are provided, with tips on creating customized reports to better view facility-level data.

Available Product Examples

Several products are available to managers and staff for review and include the following:

- Percent of respondents who are direct care providers
- The work settings that have the highest satisfaction scores
- Overall satisfaction improvement over time

Evaluation

Typically, the RN satisfaction survey reports include a downloadable PowerPoint file with the current year's analysis of findings; trends; and spreadsheets with VHA statistical significance. Facilities can view statistical significance in relation to their performance against the VA average, as well as in comparison with their own performance against the prior year's survey results. Each of the reports is provided at the VHA level, with the ability to drill down to the network or facility level. Reports can be sliced and diced to view the reports in different ways, depending on what the facility is trying to learn about its organization. Some of the ways to look at these data include by nursing role (administration, direct care, hospital support, advanced practice); nursing type (nurse practitioner, clinical specialist, certified nursing anesthetist, or RN); and work settings (acute care, continuing care, clinics, cross-settings, and interventional). In 2009, VANOD was able to obtain and program nursing unit names into the survey, allowing for a finer level of granularity in the satisfaction data.

Process Evaluation

Annually postsurvey, the survey team reviews the process and identifies issues to determine what might be done the following year so the process is smoother or concerns rectified. A timeline is shared for the next year for team review so that people have the information in their work plan. Milestones include national union notification; selection of a new marketing volunteer group and development of marketing materials; review of the prior survey for improvements needed and programming into a test environment; survey testing; and implementation and results.

National Patient Assessment Documentation Package of Templates

Background

In August 2000, the Department of Veterans Affairs (VHA) ONS tasked the future nursing workforce planning group to critically review significant aspects of the national nursing shortage and formulate strategies to ensure the ability to attract and maintain qualified nursing staff to VHA. The ONS instituted six strategic goals as part of its future strategic plan. One of these goals was technology and system development. This goal focused on the development and enhancement of systems and technology to support nursing's role in healthcare delivery models. It was essential that nursing documentation applications were integrated into the VHA computerized patient record system.

The task of the analysis group was to review the many areas of nursing documentation and recommend more efficient processes that would take advantage of future technologies and form an integrated system that reduced redundant nursing tasks documented in multiple, disparate systems. The group anticipated a major opportunity to describe a new software system that would reuse patient information entered in multiple areas of the paper and electronic record to decrease duplication of effort. There was also opportunity to develop a system that would increase patient safety by creating reminders that tell the nurse when a treatment or medication has been missed; warn the nurse of allergies; assist in ensuring the patients are prepped for procedures in a timely fashion, remind nurses of treatments and appointments; and assist in the accurate and timely documentation of care delivery. There was also opportunity to improve compliance with regulatory agencies, such as The Joint Commission. The Joint Commission requires that patient assessments and patient treatment care plans be interdisciplinary. The clinical record must be able to communicate the interdisciplinary therapy/care given to patients through multiple episodes and throughout the total continuum of care.

Through its commitment to providing identified tools for standardizing nursing documentation, ONS planned for development of a package of patient documentation templates that was comprised of three distinct templates—an admission template, a shift reassessment template, and an interdisciplinary plan of care. A template format, Delphi templates, was selected by a group of more than 48 nurses representing all aspects of nursing practice; i.e., direct care RNs, nurse executives, clinical nurse specialists, clinical nurse leaders, patient safety representatives, clinical application coordinators, researchers, etc. Multiple subcommittees were formed and identified content for the different tools. The impetus for beginning work on this package of templates was the need to be able to collect data by extraction of key data elements as a byproduct of providing care (as opposed to chart audits and Excel spreadsheets). The patient assessment documentation package of templates was accepted by the VA Office of Information and Technology as a priority product for conversion from class III (field developed) to class I (national) deployment.

The ONS patient assessment development/deployment team was chartered to use the tools available currently as a fast track work group to:

- Evaluate the new products in context of the specifications provided.
- Prepare the product for Office of Information & Technology (OI&T) deployment by making any modifications necessary to maximize compliance with the specifications, while adhering to the necessary constraints to meet OI&T parameters for the class III to class I conversion.
- Finalize content by doing the following:
  o Verify all regulatory (VHA policy, The Joint Commission, etc.) elements are included in the patient assessment.
  o Include subject matter expertise for specialty content areas.
  o Review content for evidence-based practice.
  o Verify any tools/instruments have permission from the author to be used by VHA.
- Obtain union partnership sign-off.
- Complete field-based testing and feedback cycle.
- Work with OI&T through the final release to the field.
- Design and develop a deployment tool kit that will be available prior to national release to include:
  o National communication plan
  o Facility implementation training and tool kit
  o A mechanism for ongoing field support
  o Postdeployment customer feedback processes at 6 months and at 1 year to include satisfaction with:
    □ Work flow (before and after implementation of the product)
    □ Functionality of the template
    □ Content
    □ Deployment and support
- Continue to work with OI&T through final deployment.

Scope of Use

The patient assessment will be required for inpatient admissions to acute medical, surgical, and psychiatric units. The extent of use in other specialty areas (e.g., intensive care unit) will be evaluated by the work group prior to implementation. It is expected the next body of work in this area will be to create a core data set for all areas with specialty modules for all needed points of care. The team will make final determination as to which elements of the template cannot be altered at the facility level.

Specifications for the Patient Assessment Documentation Templates

- Optimal workflow support for front line nurses—with the tools available to us today (reduce fragmentation, disruption)
- Point and click data entry with branching logic
- Functionality to save partially completed data if one is interrupted or to avoid being timed out and losing data
- Flexibility to add or delete modules
- Consideration for multistaff documentation.
- Functionality to embed discrete data elements that are:
    - Date and time stamped
    - Capable of dynamically populating downstream tools such as flow sheet, progress notes, visual graphs, etc.
    - Retrievable for local and national data extraction
- Functionality to map embedded data elements to enterprise terminology
- Functionality to extract and run the following:
    - Local reports (to be determined by the work group) for managing these groups:
        - individual patients; e.g., clinical reminders, or case management end-of-shift reports
        - whole populations; e.g., health summary
    - Extract and roll-up of national data for compiling reports for nursing processes and patient outcomes (to be determined by the work group and ONS)

- Content that meets all applicable regulatory and policy requirements
- Content that represents latest knowledge in evidence based practice
- An infrastructure so data from the patient assessment will be available for use in settings other than acute care

Steps in Development Process

The development process includes identification of a core work group for template development known as the national template team. This group was made up of:

- The ONSI project manager
- A Delphi programmer from one of the VA facilities
- Two clinical application coordinators

Refinement of Core Content

Refinement of core content involved work with the following:

- Subject matter experts for all identified specialty content (e.g., pain management, methicillin-resistant *Staphylococcus aureus* [MRSA] swabs, etc.)
- Other healthcare disciplines regarding content relative to their specialties (e.g., office of ethics, nutrition services, chaplaincy services, National Center for Patient Safety, etc.)

Identification of Pilot Sites to Test Templates in Mirror/ Test Accounts

- Twenty pilot sites were identified.
  - o Voluntary participation
  - o Testing lasted approximately 1 year
- Memorandums of understanding were signed between ONSI and each pilot facility. Signers included the facility director, the chief information resource manager, and the nurse executive.

Communication

- The plan included ongoing communication with nursing, facility, central office executive level personnel using standing meetings as well as national conferences and publications as platforms for sharing the information.

- Weekly meetings were held over the period of 1 year for pilot site resource personnel (nursing and IT representatives). The intent was for sites to provide feedback on user interface, clarity of questions, and flow of content as well as to provide opportunity for sites to ask any technical and content questions that they might have.
- Weekly meetings were held over the period of 1 year for technical team members (approximately 30 people) with OI&T personnel and enterprise system management resources. The intent was to discuss progress on the status of completion of privacy review, security plans, requirements development, 508 compliance, human factors review, etc.
- A share point site for work group of nursing and IT personnel was used.
- A go-live share point site on which to post all final documentation related to the package of templates was established.
- Ongoing communication occurred regarding the development of the templates with posting updates on the VANOD website and as agenda items on the monthly VANOD site coordinator calls.

Final Mirror Account Testing

- Testing lasted approximately 4 months.
- Testing was undertaken by the national template team, examining every conceivable scenario related to the admission and care of a patient.
- Problems not previously discovered were discovered during this intensive training.

Transfer to Office of Enterprise Development

- A completed product is turned over to the Office of Enterprise Development (under the umbrella of the Office of Information and Technology).
- A final review of the product is done by the Office of Enterprise Development team.

- Final testing in live accounts is done with sites selected from large, small, and integrated sites and from sites that have been exposed to the product and sites that have not.

Implementation

An implementation questionnaire was sent out to the VANOD site coordinators (the facility identified contacts with the VANOD) to assess the readiness of individual facilities to implement the patient assessment. The rollout of the product will occur over time, starting with smaller numbers of facilities at first and then increasing the number of facilities in each grouping if no major problems have been identified. The intent is to start rollout with sites that are in the best position to implement the templates with the least number of barriers.

Implementation teams were formed at each facility made up largely of identified superusers (at least two per shift per unit). The superusers will bear the primary responsibility for orientation of end users at each facility and will be prepared by hands-on classroom training in anticipation of this responsibility.

Evaluation

The postimplementation evaluation will be conducted at 6-month and 1-year intervals and will focus on the end user, administrative nursing staff, and technology representatives. End users will critique the new product in terms of ease of use, comparison to their last documentation tools, comprehensiveness, and clarity. Information technology staff will critique the new product in terms of setup and local installation complexity. Nursing executive/management personnel and quality staff will address the template in relation to the ability to generate valued reports from which to make administrative decisions.

Follow-Up

There is a need to have a review and update (if needed) on a yearly basis to keep the product current and representative of any changes in the system and in national clinical practice guidelines.

Summary

- The talents and skills of all team members are pivotal to IT product development and success.
- The success of projects is directly related to the leadership of stakeholders and modern IT solutions.
- IT enables staff to be more efficient and thus satisfied users.
- IT allows systems to store information and retrieve information rapidly in a global society.
- IT skill sets must be developed and used by leaders and end users for efficacy within organizations.

Reflection Question

In developing an IT product, there are several steps that must occur. Reflect on the number of individuals who may be involved and develop a strategy for buy-in by stakeholders.

References

Anantatmula, V. S. (2008). The role of technology in the project manager performance model. *Project Management Journal, 39*(1), 34–48.

California HealthCare Foundation and First Consulting Group. (2002). *Report identifies positive impact technology can have on nurse productivity and satisfaction.* Retrieved from http://www.chcf.org/media/press-releases/2002/report-identifies-positive-impact-technology-can-have-on-nurse-productivity-and-satisfaction

Cleland, D. I. (1995). Leadership and the project-management body of knowledge. *International Journal of Project Management, 13*(2), 83–88.

Karlsen, J. T., & Gottschalk, P. (2004). Factors affecting knowledge transfer in IT projects. *Engineering Management Journal, 16*(1), 3–10.

Kasvi, J. J., Vartiainen, M., & Halikari, M. (2003). Managing knowledge and knowledge competencies in projects and project organizations. *International Journal of Project Management, 21*(6), 571–582.

Prieto, I. M., & Revilla, E. (2004). Information technologies and human behaviors as interacting knowledge management enablers of the organizational learning capacity. *Internal Journal of Management Concepts and Philosophy, 1*(3), 175–197.

Runy, L. A. (2008). Information technology and nursing. *Hospitals and Health Newtworks, 8,* 1–3.

Smith, G. (2001). Making the team. *IEE Review, 47*(5), 33–36.

Thite, M. (1999). Leadership: A critical success factor in IT project management. *Proceedings of the Portland International Conference on Management and Technology (PICMET), 2,* 298–303.

Turisco, F., & Rhoads, M. S. (2008). *Equipped for efficiency: Improving nursing care through technology.* California HealthCare Foundation, Oakland, CA.

Williams, T. (2005). Assessing and moving on from the dominant project management discourse in the light of project overruns. *IEEE Transactions on Engineering Management, 52*(4), 497–508.

NINE

Developing Metrics That Support Projects and Programs

■ Mary Geary and Clista Clanton

■ Learning Objectives

1. Identify analytical and qualitative methods that support projects and programs.
2. Identify and discuss tools to assess the organization's culture and the relationship to project planning and program management.
3. Describe ways to capture project milestones.
4. Ascribe meaning to available data in designing metrics.

> "As a rule we disbelieve all the facts and theories for which we have no use."
>
> —William James

Key Terms

Evidence   Metrics

Roles

Communicator   Integrator
Decision maker   Leader
Information manager   Risk anticipator

Professional Values

Altruism   Social justice
Integrity

Core Competencies

Analyzing   Design
Appreciative inquiry   Interpersonal influence
Assessment   Presenting
Coordination   Risk
Critical thinking   Systems thinking
Data management

Introduction

In order to determine the effectiveness of any project, program, or improvement effort, there must be some type of measurement. This chapter will review a systematic approach that can be used to identify what metrics are needed to evaluate a project or program. Some projects may require data to be collected. Others may be evaluated using data that already exists within an organization. For example, in 2002, the Hospital Quality Alliance formed a voluntary collaborative for the purpose of promoting safe, quality patient care (Kurtzman, Dawson, & Johnson, 2008). The Hospital Quality Alliance has been influential in requiring hospitals to use standardized measures to evaluate care. Hospitals are required to report many of these measures to both regulatory and accrediting agencies. Much of this information is also now available to the public on various websites.

Core measures were one of the first required metrics and consist of specific evidence-based practices for certain patient diagnostic groups. Core measure data is promoted by the Centers for Medicare and Medicaid Services (CMS) as well as The Joint Commission to be a measure of a hospital's quality of patient care (Gryboski, Tilburg, & Butterick, 2009). As public pressure continues to challenge hospitals to provide safe, quality care, while containing costs, more metrics will be mandated. Many of these required measures, as well as other performance metrics typically collected by hospitals, can be useful in evaluating projects (**Table 9-1**). Therefore, before collecting any project data, one should find out what data is already being collected by various hospital departments that would be suitable for baseline and evaluation measures.

Table 9-1   Example of Hospital Metrics

Measure	Source	Hospital Department Oversight
Core measures ■ AMI ■ CHF ■ Community-acquired pneumonia ■ Surgical care improvement project ■ Children's asthma ■ Outpatient	The Joint Commission Centers for Medicaid Services (CMS)	Quality management
Nursing care sensitive measures ■ Failure to rescue ■ Pressure ulcer prevention ■ Patient falls ■ Restraint prevalence ■ Urinary catheter-associated infection	National Quality Forum	Quality management or nursing

(continues)

Table 9-1   Example of Hospital Metrics *(continued)*

Measure	Source	Hospital Department Oversight
■ Central line-associated infection ■ Ventilator-associated pneumonia		
Hospital-acquired conditions ■ Foreign object retained after surgery ■ Air embolism ■ Blood incompatibility ■ Stages III and IV pressure ulcers ■ Falls and trauma ■ Poor glycemic control ■ Catheter-associated UTI ■ Vascular-associated infection ■ Surgical site infection following coronary artery bypass graft, bariatric surgery, laparoscopic gastric restrictive surgery, orthopedic procedures (spine, neck, shoulder, elbow) ■ Deep vein thrombosis/pulmonary embolism	CMS	Quality management/ risk management
Mandatory measures ■ Medication errors ■ Adverse drug events ■ Organ donation rates ■ Sedation outcomes ■ Hand hygiene compliance ■ Resuscitation and outcomes ■ Restraint usage ■ Employee culture of safety	The Joint Commission CMS	Quality management Pharmacy Risk management

Table 9-1 Example of Hospital Metrics *(continued)*

Measure	Source	Hospital Department Oversight
Patient satisfaction	The Joint Commission	Marketing
Hospital indicators	CMS	Marketing

The likelihood that other caregivers will adopt a new hospital program or particular evidence-based practice will depend to a large extent upon the feasibility, practicality, and usefulness of the idea. Just because there is supporting research for specific patient care and treatments, it does not guarantee support from others. According to Gurses et al. (2009), compliance with implementing any evidence-based guidelines has been reported to be as low as 20%. Barriers to implementing any new practice include the lack of education among stakeholders regarding the guidelines, the lack of resources for implementation, and the lack of leadership support. The quote at the beginning of the chapter by William James suggests a fundamental barrier may be the lack of recognizing the value in making the change. So, in addition to choosing the right metrics to evaluate a program or project, one must also provide supporting measurement to demonstrate the usefulness and value to others in order to maximize the chances the project will be accepted.

Evidence-Based Practice Improvement

Evidence-based practice is the conscientious and judicious use of the current best **evidence** combined with the clinician's expertise and the patient's preferences or values in making decisions about patient care (Sackett, Rosenberg, Gray, Haynes, & Richardson, 1996). Evidence-based practice provides a framework for formulating clinical questions, searching for evidence, and critically appraising evidence to be applied in a particular practice setting. While the evidence to support decisions may come from empirical research, such as randomized controlled trials, or from descriptive data and qualitative studies, judging the strength and quality of that evidence has became a more manageable process. This is due to evidence hierarchies, ranking or grading systems for evidence-based recommendations, information tools such as evidence-based point of care databases, and evidence-based practice guidelines. However, the dissemination and adoption of evidence-based practices has not yet become a given in many practice settings, and variations in care are still widespread.

While welcoming attendees at the American Heart Association's 72nd Annual Scientific Session, the president of that organization noted that while scientific advances in the 20th century have extended life spans and eradicated many infectious diseases, there is still an epidemic of cardiovascular diseases and stroke. The organization's president observed that the issue is not in the ability to provide care, as tools and techniques such as those provided by evidence-based practice do exist, but in the ability to provide the effective application of care. So while there may be excellent scientific evidence to guide treatment, the lack of application of that evidence continues to be a problem. One suggestion made for addressing this issue was the adoption of process-improvement methods that have been used both in health care and industry and to create measurements of outcome effectiveness that will help to direct future resources and continually improve standards of care (Smaha, 2000).

Evidence-based practice improvement is a proposed model that incorporates the strengths of evidence-based practice with those of process improvement aimed at improving healthcare outcomes for patients (Levin, Perk, & Hedbäck, 1991). While there are several evidence-based nursing models that have sought to promote the adoption of evidence to guide practice in healthcare settings, they have traditionally run parallel to, rather than integrating with, practice improvement models. The strengths of practice improvement models are providing well-developed tools for implementing, evaluating, and spreading the attempted improvement efforts; understanding both the critical work processes involved in facilitating healthcare improvements and the barriers that hinder them; and fostering an environment of ongoing testing, evaluation, and learning to facilitate the adoption of the proposed changes. Since the speedy implementation of small tests of change utilized in practice improvement models have not traditionally incorporated the thorough review and appraisal of relevant research evidence for the improvements under consideration, the merging of the evidence-based practice and practice improvement models provides a more comprehensive approach to promoting the effective application of care.

The steps in the evidence-based practice improvement model are to describe the problem, formulate the clinical question, search for the evidence, appraise and synthesize that evidence, develop an AIM statement, engage in small tests of change, and then disseminate best practices. In describing the problem, it is helpful to look at both internal organizational data and information from a background literature search to frame the practice problem into a larger context. Incorporating both sets of data in forming a focused clinical question—a seemingly easy task—can prove in practice to be quite difficult. It is important to remember that not all evidence is equal and the goal is to find the highest forms of evidence as specified by evidence hierarchies. While multiple evidence hierarchies have been developed and used (Canadian Task Force on the Periodic Health Examination, 1979; Sackett, Rosenberg, Gray, Haynes, & Richardson, 1996; Cook, Stein, Krasowski, et al., 1995; Guyatt, Naylor, Juniper, Heyland, Jaeschke, & Cook, 1997; Wilson & Roof, 1997) many of these originated in the medical model and do not incorporate qualitative or other research designs. While the gold standard of individual study design has long been considered the randomized controlled trial, nursing-based hierarchies acknowledge that the concept of the randomized controlled trial gold standard could incorporate evidence that addresses dimensions such as the effectiveness, appropriateness, and feasibility of an intervention (Evans & McLeod, 2003). An example of this type of grading system is available from the Joanna Briggs Institute (JBI Levels of Evidence, 2008).

Developing an AIM statement involves establishing an operational goal and a measure of achievement to focus attention on the specific desired outcomes. For example, the statement might be, "Increase patient satisfaction scores on pain management in the burn unit by 10% in the next 6 months." Small tests of change using plan, do, study, act cycles can be implemented. The plan, do, study, act cycles provide a framework to focus the improvement and develop a plan, perform small rapid cycle tests of change, monitor the results; and continue the learning process as the results are studied. During this phase, problems can be discovered and the plan modified before a larger protocol is implemented. After the plan, do, study, act cycle is finished, disseminating the best practice within the organization on a wider scale is appropriate. After monitoring the process and outcome measures for a significant length of time (up to 2 years) to determine effectiveness and sustainability, dissemination of the best practice to a larger audience completes the evidence-based practice improvement model.

Data Management Plan

No matter what program or project is going to be evaluated, a data management plan should be developed to help guide the process of selecting the appropriate **metrics**. Using a structured approach provides a proactive guide to ensure the best measurement is initially identified and that all of the information needed for evaluation is obtained. There are six basic steps to follow, which are (1) define data needs, (2) identify data sources, (3) identify performance measures, (4) design the study, (5) retrieve the data, and (6) analyze the data.

Step One: Define Data Needs

Defining data necessary depends upon the questions to be answered. There are two general types of questions. First are quantitative questions such as "Who?" "What?" and "How many?" These questions generate numerical data that can be counted, ranked, and statistically analyzed, such as volume and frequency data. Quantitative questions are generally asked to verify something or make a prediction (Shank, 2006). Calculated means or averages can be trended over time. Medians, or the middle point of data sets, are better to use for data sets with extreme values (Brown, Aydin, & Donaldson, 2008).

The second type of question, qualitative, seeks to answer "Why?" "Why not?" and "How?" These questions are open ended to generate lots of information and gain a deeper understanding of the issue being studied. Analysis of qualitative responses is done by reviewing the responses and identifying any common themes. Qualitative questions are not as frequently used in hospitals but can often give you more timely data and be less expensive to generate (Hoff & Sutcliffe, 2006).

Using both quantitative and qualitative questions can result in a measurement set that more thoroughly evaluates a process or program. The patient satisfaction surveys used by most hospitals include both quantitative and qualitative questions. Quantitative questions ask patients to rank their response on some sort of numerical scale and address items such as level of satisfaction with nursing care, discharge planning, pain management, environmental cleanliness, and quality of food. These data can be compared and trended over time to include previous information. Most surveys also have open-ended questions that assess patients' opinions or comments. When specific comments are recurrent, then trends can be identified. Qualitative information can direct how an aspect of care might be improved or identify processes that can be replicated. Using both quantitative and qualitative data provides a holistic approach to any type of evaluation and should be used whenever possible.

Two quality-control tools that are useful in determining a specific type of questions and measurements needed for program evaluation are process flowcharts and cause-and-effect diagrams. Process flow diagrams provide a visualization of all of the steps and decision points involved in a process. The first step in creating a flow diagram is to identify the beginning and the end point of the process. An oval shape is used to represent these points. Hospital processes are usually very complex, so it is important to establish exactly what part of the process is being reviewed. The different steps within a process are represented by rectangles and appear in the order as they occur in the process. All processes have decision points that are represented in a flow diagram as diamonds. The different answers at these decision points will either lead to the next step in the process or outside the process where some other step or decision must be made before the process can continue. The number of decision points contained in a process is an indication of the process complexity. The more complex the process is, the greater the chance for breakdown or undesired outcomes.

Key measurements for analysis can be identified by reviewing the flowchart key process steps and decision points (Okes & Westcott, 2001). For example, flow diagrams can identify missing, redundant, or erroneous steps and point to improvement actions. An example of a flow diagram is in **Figure 9-1**.

A cause-and-effect diagram is useful in demonstrating the many different contributing causes of a particular problem. To construct this type of diagram, the problem (effect) is noted in the box at the right side of the chart and then major categories and subcategories that identify possible different causes are listed. Typical categories when discussing patient care problems are patient factors, staff factors, physician factors, administrative factors (policies and procedures), environmental factors, and equipment factors. A benefit of creating a cause-and-effect diagram is the brainstorming of all possible factors, which yields a broad range of possible measurements ensuring a thorough review. The cause-and-effect diagram shown is a continuation of **Figure 9-1**. After reviewing the process flow, the step of cross-matching the patient's blood specimen was identified as being a common cause for the delay. A cause-and-effect diagram was constructed to illustrate all of the possible reasons why a problem with blood cross-matching might occur (**Figure 9-2**).

Step Two: Identify Data Sources

Hospitals today, more than ever, collect a large amount of data. Much of what hospitals measure is required by the CMS to receive reimbursement for services or by The Joint Commission to demonstrate compliance with accreditation standards. The Joint Commission requires hospitals to collect data to monitor performance pertaining to restraint use, moderate sedation, adverse drug reactions, medication errors, results of

Figure 9-1   Process flow chart.

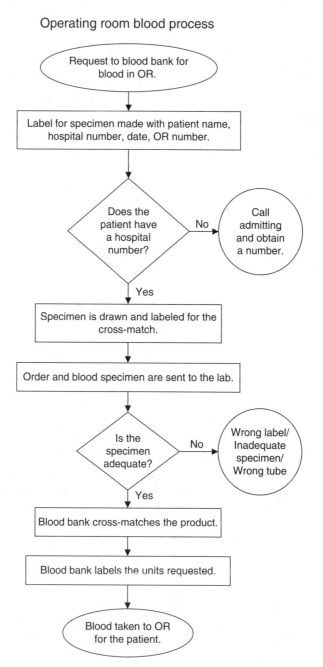

Operating room blood process

Figure 9-2   Cause-and-effect diagram.

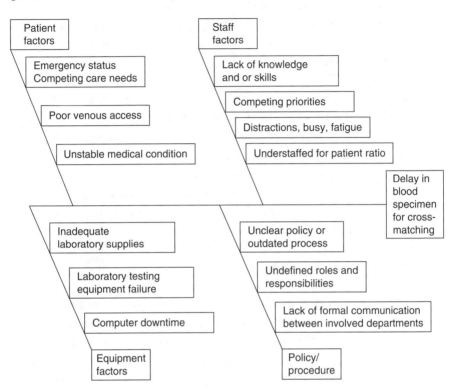

resuscitation, use of blood products, procedure complications, and preoperative and postoperative diagnosis discrepancies (The Joint Commission Hospital Standards, 2010). Hospitals also have ongoing measurements/counts of infection rates, patient falls, mortality, length of patient stay, and other metrics designed to analyze processes of care and productivity of services.

Many hospitals participate in disease-specific registries such as the Society of Thoracic Surgeons, the American College of Cardiology, and the National Surgical Quality Improvement Program. These national databases have validated measures of risk-adjusted patient outcomes for specific procedures such as coronary artery bypass surgery, percutaneous coronary interventions, and surgical care. The metrics are designed to measure evidence-based physician practices.

The most common direct measure of nursing is the National Database of Nursing Quality Indicators. This metric set was developed in 1998 by the American Nurses

Association and is currently used by more than 1,200 hospitals in the United States (Kurtzman et al., 2008). The National Database of Nursing Quality Indicators measures are based on the National Quality Forum–endorsed safe practices. The National Quality Forum's *Safe Practices for Better Healthcare* was originally released in 2003 and has been updated twice since then to incorporate current evidence and new measures (National Quality Forum, 2009). Of these measures, those most closely linked to nursing practice are referred to as nursing-sensitive measures and include nursing workforce (staffing plan and resource allocation), patient care information, order read-back and abbreviations, labeling of diagnostic studies, discharge systems, medication reconciliation, hand hygiene, surgical site infection prevention, multidrug-resistant organism prevention, venous thrombosis prevention, glycemic control, wrong-site surgery prevention, pressure ulcer prevalence, patient falls, urinary catheter-associated infections, central line catheter-associated bloodstream infections, and ventilator-associated pneumonia.

In October 2008, the CMS identified eight hospital-acquired conditions (HAC) that would cause hospitals to lose some of their Medicare reimbursement. In 2009, this list was expanded to 10 categories and reflects the National Quality Forum *Safe Practices*. These HACs were selected because evidence exists to prevent their occurrence. Many HACs are specifically linked to nursing care including stage III or IV pressure ulcers; falls and trauma; catheter-associated urinary tract infections; vascular catheter-associated infections; surgical site infections following heart surgery; bariatric procedures; and spine, neck, shoulder, and elbow procedures and glycemic control. The quality of nursing care also contributes in preventing the other HACs, including foreign object retained after surgery, air embolism, blood incompatibility, and deep vein thrombosis following knee and hip replacements.

Caution is needed when using the CMS core measures, hospital-acquired conditions data, or any data derived from administrative or coded data for analysis or conclusions. Administrative data is generated from patient classification and billing codes. Diagnostic, procedural, and complication codes are determined by medical record reviewers based on what is documented in the medical record according to established coding criteria. Thus, only what is documented in the record and interpreted by the coders will be part of the administrative database. Administrative data is not risk-adjusted for patient condition, does not include any clinical information, and can be misinterpreted in the coding process (Ko, 2009). This methodology is acknowledged in the analysis.

Step Three: Identify Performance Measures

Once the topic, specific questions, and data sources have been identified, specific measures are determined. Three types of measures are used, including structural, process, and outcome measures. Structural measures refer to the attributes of a healthcare organization and how it is organized to deliver care. Examples of structural measures include staffing ratios, patient skill mix, and procedure volumes. These measures are typically easy to access from administrative databases and do not require manual data collection. In the past, measuring surgical volumes or specific patient program enrollment volumes has been used as a measure of an organization's quality of care. However, the significance of the relationship between volumes to outcomes has only been demonstrated for a few procedures (Ko, 2009). Structural measures can be indirectly related to both process and outcome measures. Having a combination of all three types of measures can be useful in evaluating different aspects of a process (**Table 9-2**). Aiken (2001) examined the relationship between nursing staffing ratios (structural measures) and the use of evidence-based care practices (process measures) as well the staff ratios' relationships with the quality of patient outcomes (outcome measures), which provided much of the rationale for hospitals to link these three variables together when trying to improve patient care.

Process measures typically evaluate whether processes are being followed as designed. They can measure specific steps of a process or an entire process and usually fall into categories of financial, utilization, compliance, disease specific, and satisfaction with care (Lighter, 2011). The CMS core measures are all process measures designed to determine the frequency of specific evidence-based practices. The CMS requires measuring processes to facilitate optimal patient outcomes that should occur. The underlying assumption is that if the core measure practices for pneumonia patients, for example, are instituted, then a patient with pneumonia will have a greater chance of having a positive outcome. However, many factors and processes can influence patients' outcomes, so inferences regarding any causal relationships should be made with caution. The patient's other health risks may affect his or her recovery, infection prevention practices of the patient's caregivers could cause the patient to develop a nosocomial infection, and the skill of the cardiologist can determine the success of any cardiac interventions. Therefore, measuring outcomes such as complications, infections, and mortality are also important in the overall evaluation of a program or project.

Table 9-2 Structure, Process, and Outcome Measures for Cardiac Catheterization

Measure	Jan	Feb	Mar	April	May	June	July	Aug	Sept	Oct	Nov	Dec	Total
Volume (structural measures)													
No. of catheters													
No. of diagnostic													
No. of interventional													
Process measures													
Closure device used (Y/N)													
Fluoro time													
No. of stents													
Complications (Outcome measures)													
No. of hematomas													
No. of required transfusions													
No. requiring surgery													

No. requiring unplanned intervention										
No. of acute closures										
No. of closures w/in 6 mos										
No. of codes E—expired; S—survived										
No. of balloon pumps used										
No. of AMI following catheterization										
No. of deaths										

AMI, acute myocardial infarctions.

Outcome measures are used to determine the effectiveness of processes. Two types of outcomes are common in health care—operational and clinical outcomes. Both are important in program evaluation. Operational outcomes measure how well a nonclinical process is performing and include financial data, environmental inspection data, patient satisfaction with food, and cleanliness. Clinical outcome measures are specific to a clinical condition or the result of specific treatment and care. Many national registries such as the National Surgical Quality Improvement Program provide clinical outcome data that is risk adjusted for each patient according to comorbidities and other identified related factors (Ko, 2009). Risk-adjusted outcome data are a more accurate measure of how well a treatment or process is working.

There are many valid and reliable assessment tools that can be used to define concepts to be measured. For example, when measuring patients' risk for skin breakdown, using the Braden scale to define high risk gives a specific definition and ensures an objective, consistent measurement. One should not assume to know the meaning as many concepts can be subjectively defined. For example, measuring a patient's level of pain will vary from patient to patient and could vary based on what specific type of pain measurement scale is used to quantify the pain. A level-5 pain may be the most severe pain on a 1–5 scale but moderate pain on a 1–10 scale. Another example is the different definitions of fall rates; some include patient and visitor falls while others include only patients. Performance measures must be defined before measuring and preferably using definitions that have already been validated and used in the nursing literature.

Performance measures need to be reliable and valid. Reliability is defined as the extent to which the data generated are consistent with what is being measured and the variable of interest is measured the same way in each participant (Polit & Beck, 2004). Performance measures are said to be valid when they measure what is intended to be studied. Poor validity can occur if the measure is indirectly linked to a concept or if the variables are not clearly defined.

Step Four: Design the Study

The study design is determined by the focus of the project or program and the specific aspects being evaluated. However, some basic concepts are defining the population of interest and determining the sample size. For example, if the project focuses on preventing urinary tract infections in hospitalized patients, the population of interest would be all patients who have an indwelling catheter. In a large hospital, it may not be possible to include all patients so a representative sample would be needed. Current minimum sample size is 5% or 30 items, whichever is greater (Williams & Geary, 1997). If the population is less than 30, every case needs to be reviewed.

Step Five: Retrieve the Data

Many projects fail because data retrieval is not systematically planned, resulting in wrong or incomplete data being obtained, leading to inability to analyze or measure the concept of interest (Lighter, 2011). Systematically planning the retrieval of data includes deciding where and how to access data that is already being collected, or, if data is not already available, deciding who will collect the data, how data will be gathered, and the specific time period for the collection. This is especially critical to do if more than one person is doing the data retrieval to ensure consistent methods. Data collection tools are helpful in ensuring consistency in data retrieval (**Table 9-3**) Data can come from a variety of sources and retrieval methods can include observation, medical record review, surveys, and interviews. The information needed will determine the best source of the data; the more direct measure of a concept the stronger the analysis. For example, observing a practice is a more accurate measure than reviewing a chart for documentation of the practice. The ease of obtaining data is also an important factor and can sometimes cause one to use a more indirect measure of the concept.

It is also necessary to decide on the time period for measurement. Most administrative data, such as core measures, are retrospective measurements. Advantages of retrospective data collection include convenience and use of administrative databases, which allow for quick and large-scale evaluations to be done. Examples of retrospective data retrieval include using administrative data based on specific codes, medical record abstractions from previous hospitalizations and posthospital/ procedure surveys. A disadvantage of retrospective data is there is delay of sometimes several months between when a process change or improvement action is implemented and when the retrospective data will be available to analyze for any effects. Therefore, retrospective data is not best for projects of an urgent nature needing immediate review.

Concurrent measurement refers to real time data collection; the length of time for data collection depends on the amount of data needed to reach the appropriate sample size. The disadvantage of concurrent measurement is it takes more time and effort to collect the data. The advantages, however, are that data can be trended

Table 9-3   Patient Safety Liaisons Data Collection Form

Patient Safety Unit-Based Rounds

Unit: _____ Month/Year _____ Completed by: _____

Issue—Mark Each as Yes; No; n/a	MR No.	MR No.	MR No.	MR No.	MR No.
Patient Interview and Observation Items:					
1. The patient was encouraged not to leave his/her clinical area and if he or she does, to have signed release in chart.					
2. The correct armband is on the patient.					
3. Ask the patient if new caregivers are asking him/her to state his/her full name and checking his/her armband prior to giving him/her medications or blood.					
4. Patients at a high risk for falling have on a yellow armband and a fall leaf placed on the door.					
Medications/IV solutions					
5. IV medications are labeled with correct patient name, time IV hung, and ordered drug/dose if not already labeled.					
6. The IV site is dated, timed, and changed every 72 hours.					
7. The IV pump library is in use for heparin, insulin, and chemotherapy agents.					
8. A medication reconciliation form is completed on admission.					
9. PCA pumps have a booklet and a warning label for patient to push only.					

Table 9-3   Patient Safety Liaisons Data Collection Form *(continued)*

Patient Safety Unit-Based Rounds

Unit: _____ Month/Year _____ Completed by: _____

Issue—Mark Each as Yes; No; n/a	MR No.	MR No.	MR No.	MR No.	MR No.
Chart review					
10. Documentation of read-back of orders has been done.					
11. Documentation of read-back of critical values, tests, and procedure results has been done.					
12. Allergies are documented on all required forms.					
13. Signature indicating informed consent has been obtained for any surgical or invasive bedside procedure and matches the procedure on the order or postprocedure note.					
14. All invasive procedures have a final time out entered.					
15. No "do not use" abbreviations are found in the progress notes or orders. If so, list which ones (write "none" or the specific abbreviations used).					
17. The Morse fall scale is recorded on the graphics according to the patient's risk level.					
18. The Braden scale is recorded on the initial assessment sheet according to the patient's risk level.					

(continues)

Table 9-3   Patient Safety Liaisons Data Collection Form *(continued)*

Patient Safety Unit-Based Rounds

Unit: _____ Month/Year _____ Completed by: _____

Issue—Mark Each as Yes; No; n/a	MR No.	MR No.	MR No.	MR No.	MR No.
Observation measure (actual number of behaviors observed/total number behaviors possible)					
19. The number of times hand hygiene was done/number of times hand hygiene should have been done (before and after patient care, staff breaks, eating, etc.).	/	/	/	/	/
20. Ask the nurse whether patient transporters are initiating the "ticket to ride."					
21. Refrigerator logs are being completed to document temperature checks.					
22. Code carts are being checked and documented daily.					

MR, medical record.

during this collection time and any issues can be promptly identified and addressed. With retrospective data, any issues have already occurred, and there is no opportunity to intervene at the time of occurrence.

Step Six: Analyze the Data

The last step of the data management plan is to analyze the measurement data to determine any necessary changes. Data analysis is often the weakest step and is frequently inadequately performed. There are some simple statistical tools that can assist in analyzing the effect of an action or the success of a project. Several different types of charts can easily be constructed using standard computer programs. The type of chart needed will depend on the measures and the information needing analysis.

One of the most basic charts designed to identify trends in the variables is a run chart. Run charts are line graphs that display data over time and can show whether there has been a change in the performance after an intervention is implemented. One process or several can be shown on the same chart if the data is being analyzed for comparisons in trends (**Figure 9-3**). This line (or run) in the chart depicts the process variation. All processes have variation that is either part of the process itself (common cause variation) or due to external influences (special cause variation) (Lighter, 2011). Being able to recognize the special cause variation is important especially when analyzing for effects from an intervention. Run charts typically have the time interval on the horizontal axis and the variable being measured on the vertical axis. The data is plotted over time and variation is evaluated. Two special cause trends are runs and shifts. Runs mean there is a continual increase or decrease seen for six data points in a row, and shifts cause data points to all fall above or below the average or centerline. Runs and shifts need to be analyzed further in order to determine the cause of the variation.

Control charts are run charts that include the process parameters of mean and standard deviation calculated from the process data itself. These parameters make

Figure 9-3 Run chart comparing two processes: Rapid response team calls and codes.

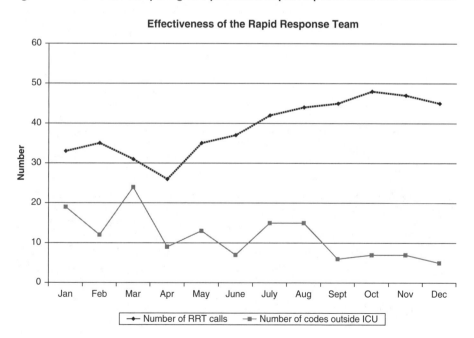

the centerline (mean) and the upper and lower control limits. The control limits are determined by adding or subtracting the standard deviation to or from the mean. Control limits can be set as one, two, or three standard deviations above and below the process mean depending on what is being measured and how much variance is acceptable. The more standard deviations used, the larger the control limits and the more variation is accepted before the process is said to need additional analysis. So if the control chart is trending serious patient issues (mortalities, infections, etc.), the control limits would best be set at one or two standard deviations so only minimum occurrences would be tolerated. Both the run chart and control chart are useful tools to use when analyzing data over time to determine if a process is performing as designed or if a change has occurred—whether intentional, unintentional, positive, or negative. If data stays within the control limits, the process is stable. The process is unstable when data points are found to be outside of the control limits and further investigation is needed to determine the special cause(s) of the variation. In the control chart example (**Figure 9-4**), there are 3 months when the number of patients leaving the emergency department before they are seen were outside the control limits. All three of these months should be further reviewed to determine any specific causes or common factors.

Figure 9-4   Control chart with mean, standard deviations.

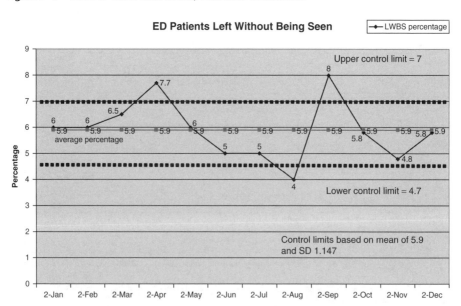

Two types of bar charts that are useful for analyzing the frequency or pattern of the data over a time period are the histogram and the Pareto charts. A histogram is used to determine if the process has a normal distribution (**Figure 9-5**). Data is said to be bell shaped or normally distributed when the most frequent data appears within the center of the graph with equal data points appearing on either side (Okes & Westcott, 2001). An abnormal distribution or shape indicates that the process is not performing as designed and additional review is needed.

A Pareto chart is a bar chart that shows the frequency of measures. This type of graph is based upon the Pareto principle, which states that 80% of the process variation, or cause of a problem, is based on 20% of the variables (Okes & Westcott, 2001). The bars in the Pareto chart are ranked in descending frequency with the variables listed on the horizontal axis and frequency on the vertical axis. In **Figure 9-6**, the most frequent cause identified for calling the rapid response team is patients having hypotension. Being able to make this analysis helps direct any additional information needed to identify any common factors contributing to these patients developing hypotension.

Figure 9-5   Example of a normal distribution histogram.

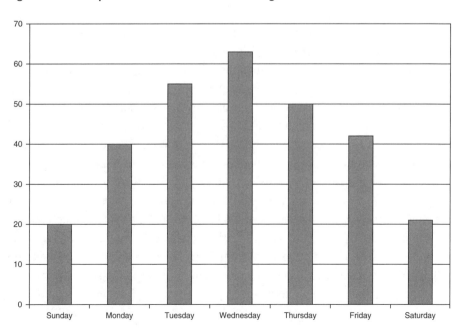

Figure 9-6   Pareto chart showing most frequent to least frequent reason for RRT calls.

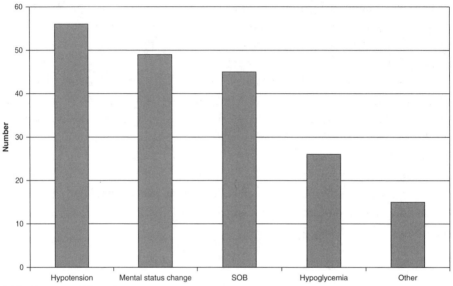

Frequency of Reasons for RRT Calls

SOB, shortness of breath.

The last chart that is helpful in analyzing data is a scatter diagram. Scatter diagrams are useful in determining if there is a correlation between two variables. A positive correlation is indicated when there is an upward slope found among the data points. A negative correlation is seen when the pattern slopes downward, which occurs when one variable's increase correlates with the other variable's decrease. When there is not an identifiable pattern found, the scatter diagram is interpreted as showing there is no correlation between the two variables. A positive or negative correlation does not necessarily mean there is a direct cause-and-effect relationship between the two variables. There is also no way to determine the strength of the correlation from a scatter diagram. Additional measurement would be needed for that type of analysis. The first step involved in constructing a scatter diagram is to determine the variables and the type of relationship being investigated (cause/cause; cause/effect). Next, obtain paired data for the two variables and place the cause on the horizontal axis and the effect on the vertical axis. Finally, plot the data and check for any patterns. Patterns are interpreted as positive correlations, no correlations, or negative correlations, as shown in **Figure 9-7**.

Figure 9-7   Different correlations found in scatter diagrams.

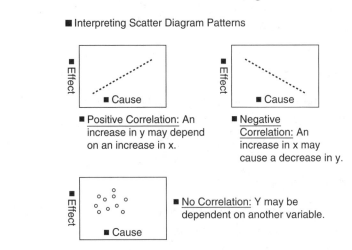

It is important to have a data management plan to determine the measures needed to support and evaluate any project or new program. Many different hospital departments perform ongoing measurement to evaluate different processes and outcomes. Some of these measures are suitable to use to evaluate and analyze new aspects of care, but often additional data is needed to be able to do a true analysis of an issue. If additional measures are needed, then the most direct measurement of the concept should be considered. Also, there are always new questions raised when analyzing a project or program. Using the appropriate statistical process tools will contribute to a comprehensive analysis and guide decision making.

Summary

- A systematic approach is requisite for project and program evaluation.
- Core measure data are the markers of an organization's quality of care.
- Evidence-based practice improvements are based on a series of rigorous outcomes and research that have been sustainable.
- Data management plans guide the process for selecting metrics.
- Data management plans determine the measures needed to support and evaluate any project or program.

- Decisions are best made when based on data.
- Several different charts and graphs can be developed to track, trend, and illustrate quality outcomes.

Reflection Questions

1. What is the relevance of building project milestones in project plans?
2. What is the best strategy/approach to assessing an organization's readiness for a change project? How can this be measured?

Learning Activities

1. Review quality data for one unit and compare to a like unit. Identify the differences and draw conclusions on similarities or/and differences.
2. Compare and contrast different ways that quality data can be visually displayed.

References

Aiken, L. (2001). An international perspective on hospital nurses' work environments: The case for reform. *Policy, Politics & Nursing Practice, 2*(4), 255–263.

Brown, D., Aydin, C., & Donaldson, N. (2008). Quartile dashboards: Translating large data sets into performance improvement priorities. *Journal for Healthcare Quality, 30*(6), 18–30.

Cook, E. H., Stein, M. A., Krasowski, M. D., Cox, N. J., Olkon, D. M., Kieffer, J. E., et al. (1995). Association of attention-deficit disorder and the dopamine transporter gene. *American Journal of Human Genetics, 56*(4), 993–998.

Evans, W. E., & McLeod, H. L. (2003). Pharmacogenomics—Drug disposition, drug targets, and side effects. *NEJM, 348*(6), 538–549.

Gryboski, A., Tilburg, J., & Butterick, J. (2009). Quality buckets: An innovative tool for complying with healthcare mandates. *Journal for Healthcare Quality, 31*(6), 3–7.

Gurses, A., Murphy, D., Martinez, E., Berenholtz, S., & Pronovost, P. (2009). A practical tool to identify and eliminate barriers to compliance with evidence-based guidelines. *The Joint Commission Journal on Quality and Patient Safety, 35*(10), 526–535.

Guyatt, G. H., Naylor, C. D., Juniper, E., Heyland, D. K., Jaeschke, R., & Cook, D. J. (1997). Users' guides to the medical literature. XII. How to use articles about health-related quality of life. *JAMA, 277*(15), 1232–1237.

Hoff, T., & Sutcliffe, K. (2006). Studying patient safety in health care organizations: Accentuate the qualitative. *The Joint Commission Journal on Quality and Patient Safety, 32*(1), 5–15.

The Joint Commission. (2010). *2010 Comprehensive accreditation manual for hospitals: The official handbook (CAMH).* Oak Brook, IL: The Joint Commission Resources.

Ko, C. (2009, November/December). Measuring and improving surgical quality. *Patient Safety and Quality Healthcare,* 36–41. Retrieved from http://www.psqh.com/novemberdecember-2009/311-measuring-and-improving-surgical-quality.html

Kurtzman, E., Dawson, E., & Johnson, J. (2008). The current state of nursing performance measurement, public reporting and value-based purchasing. *Policy, Politics & Nursing, 9*(3), 181–190.

Lighter, D. E. (2011). *Advanced performance improvement in health care: Principles and methods.* Sudbury, MA: Jones and Bartlett.

Levin, L. A., Perk, J., & Hedbäck, B. (1991). Cardiac rehabilitation—a cost analysis. *Journal of Internal Medicine, 230*(5), 427–434.

National Quality Forum. (2009). *Safe practices for better healthcare: 2009 update* (a consensus report). Washington, DC: Author.

Okes, D., & Westcott, R. (2001). *The certified quality manager handbook.* Milwaukee, WI: American Society for Quality Press Publications.

Polit, D., & Beck, C. (2004). *Nursing research: Principles and methods* (7th ed.). Philadelphia: Lippincott Williams & Wilkins.

Sackett, D. L., Rosenberg, W., Gray, J. A., Haynes, R. B., & Richards, W. S. (1996). Evidence-based medicine: What it is and what it isn't [Editorial]. *British Medical Journal, 312*(7023), 71–72.

Shank, G. (2006). *Qualitative research* (2nd ed.). Upper Saddle River, NJ: Pearson.

Smaha, L. (2000). Message from China. *Circulation,* 102, e67–e68.

Williams, T. P., & Geary, M. E. (1997). *Improving nursing performance.* Chicago: Precept Press.

Wilson, R. B., & Roof, D. M. (1997). Respiratory deficiency due to loss of mitochondrial DNA in yeast lacking the frataxin homologue. *Nature Genetics, 16*(4), 352–357.

TEN

Measuring the Value of Projects Within Organizations

■ Michael R. Bleich

■ Learning Objectives

1. Describe ways to assign value to a project.
2. Discuss the relevance of measuring project value.
3. Discuss mechanisms to communicate the value of a project.

"Quality in a product or service is not what the supplier puts in. It is what the customer gets out and is willing to pay for. A product is not quality because it is hard to make and costs a lot of money, as manufacturers typically deliver. This is incompetence. Customers pay only for what is of use to them and gives them value. Nothing else constitutes quality."

—Peter F. Drucker

Key Terms

Evidence   Information management

Roles

Communicator   Information manager
Decision maker   Leader
Integrator   Risk anticipator

Professional Values

Altruism   Social justice
Integrity

Core Competencies

Assessment   Interpersonal influence
Coordination   Leadership
Critical thinking/appreciative inquiry Management
Design   Risk reduction
Emotional intelligence   Systems thinking

Introduction

When an organization undertakes a project, it is typically for a specific intention that aligns with its mission and vision. Resources, usually constrained, are invested and used, which means that these same resources are being shifted from other parts of the organization for use by the project undertaking. This simple frame belies the essence of this chapter—that value must be attained and measured to ensure that the resources did, in fact, advance the organization's mission and vision and that the investment of resources into the project yielded value to the organization's stakeholders, who are, notably in health care, those who require clinical service.

Measuring value is difficult both conceptually and practically. First, measurement requires the use of information, usually drawn from databases but often collected specifically for a project, based on the anticipated outcomes of the project. The information collected must be informative, meaning that a predesigned plan for its use has been determined. If it informs, then it must also be relevant to the project and sensitive so that it measures real differences in the project's anticipated impact. Further, information must be unbiased and comprehensive enough to capture the scope and magnitude of the project, such that the integrity of the project's impact is real. Measuring the impact of a project also requires timely information. Additionally, how that information is stored and maintained must be considered so that impact can be measured throughout the project's duration. In project management, information must be performance targeted to the goals and objectives of the project, collected in a uniform manner, and, importantly, cost effective and possible to obtain. These attributes, as per Austin (1979), have been a foundation for project management and quality improvement changes that have served my own leadership practice over time.

The next challenge is how to capture value. Drucker's quote to open this chapter suggests that value is different from cost and that it serves to meet the perceptual needs of a stakeholder. Value is expressed by first knowing the stakeholder's interest. In the case of a project that influences organizational efficiencies, this may be measured in time saved, simplifying a complex task, replacing a way of working that is distasteful with one that is opposite, supplanting one method for another, and the like. There may be dimensions of cost effectiveness, job autonomy, and other factors. The project manager must be clear about the stakeholder's needs and wants in order to form the baseline for comparison of outcomes. Similarly, if the project impacts patient care, then the patient's perceptions must be considered. Will the project create ease of access to care? Or will it provide for symptom management, influence quality of life, diminish pain or discomfort, or reduce the advancement of disease to a higher stage of chronicity? The project leader must be clear about the aim of the project and establish this from a value perspective. As stated earlier, measuring value is complex and requires considerable forethought and design (Fitzgerald, 2004).

If it is not already apparent, the project manager will play multiple roles in measuring the value of projects within organizational settings. Measuring the value of impact in any project must be considered even before the onset of the project. The project manager must understand the genesis of the project, especially when a project is delegated as an opportunity that his or her boss has for him or her. What were the organizational dynamics that led to the project? What are the strategic and operational impacts desired from the project? Who are the affected stakeholders? What, in the creation of change, is going to be lost and what is going to be gained as a result of the project? The role of leadership comes into play by venturing into the unknown. The role of manager is executed by guiding the project through a defined process. But additional roles germane to this chapter are also relevant: The project manager must be strategic and must function as a planner, the **communicator** (which includes being a sleuth in order to understand people, processes, and structures that influence the project), a data analyst, and even a database administrator. Value, then, based on stakeholder expectations, may be expressed in terms of time saved, cost, convenience/access, simplicity of use, and more.

Aligning Metrics with Project Aims

Projects vary in terms of the magnitude and scope of the change, the stakeholders involved, and the degree of linearity or complexity associated with the approach taken to manage the project. **Table 10-1** provides a useful framework for examining a project's level of complexity (Berger, 2005).

Table 10-1 Project Characteristics as a Precursor to Metric Selection

Simple Project	Mid-Range Project	Complex Project
Stakeholders are limited to a select few, often with readily aligned values and needs.	Stakeholders are modest in number and cross boundaries within an organizational setting where values and needs are similar.	Stakeholders are large in number or are of varying disciplines with often disparate values and needs.
The project is primarily linear with clearly defined outcomes targeted at individuals and groups.	The project is both linear and nonlinear in that the outcomes extend to influence behaviors that are less defined and that focus at the group level of attainment.	The project is primarily nonlinear with less defined structure and the outcomes cannot be clearly defined and are aimed at social change.

Table 10-1   Project Characteristics as a Precursor to Metric Selection

Simple Project	Mid-Range Project	Complex Project
The project manager retains the ability to oversee and control each aspect of project activities.	The project manager works with a team to oversee and provide general direction while the project unfolds and morphs to meet unanticipated needs.	The project manager does not exist in one individual, but rather extends to intersecting groups, all of whom share a common aim and multiple strategies emerge to shape the direction of the project.
Metrics are simple to retrieve from existing data and can be readily observed or collected; feedback loops are easy to define and are often from a single source.	Metrics are retrieved from multiple data sources and may require development beyond what is available, with feedback loops required from multiple sources.	Metrics are retrieved from large databases and public opinion and must capture the multiple interests within divergent populations and stakeholders.
Metrics are focused on project completion and simple outcomes.	Metrics are focused on organizational impact and more complex outcomes, beyond project completion to project impact.	Metrics are focused on social change with complex social outcomes.
The value to measure is tied to a few defined concepts within a narrow range.	The value to measure is tied to multiple concepts within a broad organizational range.	The value to measure is tied to social concepts that cross organizational boundaries.

An example of a simple project might be the introduction of a product that is available at the point of care to encourage hand hygiene. The aim of the project has a defined location (bedside), a defined targeted audience (bedside caregivers), and a targeted aim (nosocomial infection reduction or prevention). As simple as this might seem, the project leader must consider what to measure. Should we measure hand-washing compliance using the product? Should we measure changes in nosocomial infection rates? Will we measure the impact of the product in real time or retrospectively? Is there an existing database from which to draw information? Does one need to be created? Will we sample for outcomes or include the entire population? When is the best time to collect the data to represent the results with integrity and to reduce risk? Who will collect the data and how will data collection be coordinated? From this example, there are many clues to indicate that the complexities of measuring value are endless.

Case Study Application

A project manager has been appointed based on a community desire to be more heart healthy. The hospital responded favorably to this community request, which emanated from several organizations including the YMCA, the statewide affiliate of the American Heart Association, and civic leaders whose concern was a healthy workforce. A cardiovascular nurse leader was selected by the hospital CEO to lead the hospital's efforts to make a huge impact on cardiovascular health. The project aims included assuring that exercise was available to all age groups year-round, having one or more citizens trained in CPR reside on every city block, and placing a defibrillator device in all public buildings with an occupancy of 75 or more people. Note that, fortunately, the project aims were all measurable, which is not always the case!

The nurse leader charged with this project had a number of complex design challenges to think through, beginning with a willing spirit and strong personal values that the project was a good thing! Using Table 10-1 as a reference, the nurse determined that there were components of the project that could be subdivided and that crossed over all project levels from simple to complex. The leader recognized that the project had dimensions that addressed social justice and that there was an altruistic component to it. **Evidence** about cardiovascular disease supported the project and could be used for ideas about measuring the project's impact. Evidence that did not already exist also needed to be gathered. The following questions needed to be answered: How many establishments exist that accommodate 75 or more people? How many have automatic external defibrillators? Further, how many city blocks exist and where do the city limits end? Does the charter really mean city blocks, or should suburbs be included? What are the ramifications if they are not included? What is the anticipated risk of limiting the project to the city? How does one define *exercise*? What are socially acceptable norms relating to exercise given weather conditions and public safety issues? How will the communities of interest value and accept the risk associated with exercise or the lack thereof?

Only when these and similar questions were answered could an effective metric design and **information management** plan emerge. Systems thinking was needed by the nurse leader to understand the interrelated components of the project and to recognize which parts of the project had linear, systematic, and predictable components to them versus other aspects of the project that targeted larger social and policy issues. In a brainstorming session around metrics, the following suggestions emerged:

- We could collect data on satisfaction with CPR training.
- We could count the number of individuals who exercise on a regular basis.
- We could look at the number of heart-related procedures that are performed at the local hospital and see if those go down.
- We could look at claims databases to check for cardiac risk factors.
- We could mandate that vending machines have their food choices altered to include healthy alternatives and count the changes.
- We could count the number of people who attend a health fair and have their blood pressure taken.
- We could restrict public smoking because of its link to heart disease and monitor heart disease occurrences.
- We could count the number of new exercise programs that are held in public places, including long-term-care facilities.

If you were going to use this list, how useful would it be to you? Which data are tied to simple, mid-range, and complex social change? How accessible is the information suggested? Is it performance targeted? Is it new or existing data? How does it tie to the project objectives set forth? How do the metrics suggested integrate with the project? What would you change?

Principles of Project Evaluation Methods

Project evaluation is an effort to measure the impact of project-based change. The value proposition to be measured is derived from the stakeholders themselves, which often are diverse. One stakeholder (e.g., a shareholder) may have a singular interest in profit. Another stakeholder (e.g., a patient) may have an interest in access, cost, and quality. Regulators may want adherence to a defined set of standards. Many projects evolve from quality improvement initiatives, where metrics are a close "cousin" to project management metrics. In fact, the principles of developing metrics for quality improvement serve as a substantive guide for project evaluation (Berger, 2005; Lloyd, 2004).

In order to adequately meet the needs of the stakeholders, the project manager (note that this is not a formal title but rather a temporary job assignment, such as in the case study) bears responsibility for measuring the impact of project objectives or aims. These objectives should readily be aligned with the organization's mission and purpose if the level of change is targeted within an institutional setting. But some projects extend to multiple settings and are therefore more complex for determining a single value proposition. Insurance companies may have a desire to provide different health education, for instance, than what is desired by a provider–patient relationship. These differences must be accounted for in complex changes.

Some researchers compare project evaluation methods as being closely aligned with the field of program evaluation. As defined by Fink, program evaluation is a

> diligent investigation of a program's characteristics and merits. Its purpose is to provide information on the effectiveness of projects so as to optimize the outcomes, efficiency, and quality of health care. Evaluations can analyze a program's structure, activities, and organization and examine its political and social environment. They can also appraise the achievements of a project's goals and objectives and the extent of its impact and costs. (1993, p. 2)

Fink differentiated project and program evaluation from other types of research in that its major task is to judge a program's merits. She defined a meritorious program/project as one that has "worthy goals, achieves its standards of effectiveness, provides benefits to its participants, fully informs its participants of potential risks of participation, and does no harm" (1993, p. 2). Developing value metrics in an organizational context, then, can relate to measuring program objectives and activities, program outcomes, and program impact.

The methods used to capture data include both quantitative and qualitative strategies. As used here, quantitative methods include approaches that measure impact through mechanisms such as data retrieval from existing administrative and national databases, economic cost-effectiveness determination, surveys measuring perceptions, and targeted research instruments that measure patient, family, and societal outcomes that align with the project objectives and aims. Examples of quantitative data include selecting metrics from the following:

■ Clinical/epidemiologic databases, such as those contained in disease registries or through epidemiologic surveys (Johantgen, 2005)
■ Administrative claims data at the organization or state level (Johantgen, 2005)
■ Sociodemographic data, such as that available through census reports and state-level vital statistics records
■ Patient satisfaction data, such as that available through proprietary databases at the institutional level (Hayes, 2008)
■ National Data on Nursing Quality Indicators (NDNQI) data, applied at the institutional level (Montalvo, 2007; Trossman, 2006)
■ Marketing data that specifies lifestyle and other useful population practices

Similarly, qualitative data provide rich context for project impact. These data are available through the following:

■ Focus groups with project-oriented aims
■ Appreciative inquiry/story-telling methods aligned with stakeholder groups (Whitney & Trosten-Bloom, 2003)
■ Internet and social networking approaches to capture context

Information Dissemination: Roles and Responsibilities for Communication

The project manager has the ultimate responsibility to ensure that the impact of project implementation is reflected in useful ways to stakeholder groups. As early data are collected, the dissemination of information is critical to the stabilization of the project. Those engaged in the change need and want feedback on how the project is progressing. While the full impact of change may be unknown in the early stages of data collection, it does provide motivation toward meeting project aims and objectives. Chapter 9 gives greater detail to the dissemination process.

Face-to-face communication is helpful, but when it comes to data presentation, it simply is not enough. The accountable project manager displays data using charts, survey tools, graphs, and other means to fully reflect the impact of the project during its implementation and at the conclusion of the intervention, and continues through to monitor postintervention effectiveness and restabilization. Today, electronic support of data presentation and analysis underscores the need to be transparent in all facets of program accountability.

Rarely do projects turn out exactly as planned. If the right metrics are selected, namely, those that show sensitivity to the project aims and objectives, and if the data are reliably collected and displayed, then variation will occur from the plan. This does not mean failure of the project but, rather, presents an opportunity for the project leader and stakeholder groups to "torture the data" as John Ruskin was quoted as saying, such that meaning emerges from the data. In other words, data themselves do not signify success or failure of a project. Only collective meaning and an eye toward improvement derive a project's success. Too often, project managers feel the obligation to measure that which appears to denote success rather than capture what is successful—or not—about a project.

The presentation of feedback through quantitative and qualitative data presents the opportunity for the project leader to anticipate risk, integrate findings with lived reality, communicate a sense of purpose to the stakeholders, and design plans for improving the project past its due date and into the fabric of the work of the organization.

Especially in the case of projects that lead to system change, the use of statistical process control charts helps to determine the impact of the change and resets the new and improved standard, such that variation can be identified as that which is created by the system change itself (known as common cause variation) or as a major aberrancy that rests outside of the system change (special cause variation) (Deming, 1986). These techniques, used in quality improvement, are critical to help determine whether a changed system is performing in a desirable manner and quickly draw attention to special causes that are not related to the change itself. Although outside of the scope of this chapter, statistical process control tools should be within the realm of project managers to aid in decision making and direction setting (Carey & Lloyd, 2001).

Lastly, it is important to portray the effects of change to stakeholder groups. A final report, a summary e-mail, a closure event to mark achievements, or the presence of run charts with notes attached to denote accomplishments are all mechanisms that can be employed to tell the story of the value that the project brought to the organization, its stakeholders, and others who evaluate the organization, such as external regulators, public constituency groups, and the like. Today, nurse leaders are not present often enough in the boardroom to discuss change, but a well-educated project leader, with the right tools for communication and data presentation, should be present at the venue to advance patient care and to inform others of the contributions of nursing and other healthcare professionals.

Tools of the Trade

In project management, inexpensive statistical process control software is readily available. Some basic procedures can be performed with an Excel spreadsheet. When these tools are used, the process changes that have occurred can be monitored for common cause and special cause variation, as described previously. The control chart that emanates from statistical process control powerfully documents change and variability (Kelley, 1999).

Similarly, graphic presentation of data is useful, particularly when it can be modeled in a dashboard style of presentation. A dashboard presentation compares and contrasts metrics into a single document, such that patient outcomes, staff performance, economic data, and risk data, for example, can be studied as a set, aiding decision making by displaying that one variable (e.g., cost savings) is not working against other variables (e.g., patient satisfaction). This is another important tool for decision making and evaluation (Nelson, 1995).

Summary

- Value is about knowing the specific stakeholder wants and needs related to the project. These can vary widely, but they often include access to service, cost-effective delivery of service, and satisfaction with the project's outcomes.
- Metrics is the art and science of measuring value. Metrics must be informative, relevant, unbiased and comprehensive, action oriented, performance targeted, and cost effective.
- Projects vary in complexity and the metrics will vary accordingly.

- Metrics can include both quantitative and qualitative data; whereas the former provides information about specific points of achievement, the latter provides context. They are complementary.
- Project leaders are accountable for a fair and honest representation of the project and should be prepared to reveal progress toward the aims, as well as unanticipated outcomes, both positive and negative.
- Project leaders should use decision science tools, such as those associated with statistical process control and dashboard mapping to represent their work and to adapt projects as needed.
- Data should support the project from before the onset of the project through to project stabilization, sometime after the project's impact has settled into the culture of work.

Suggested Readings

Maeda, J. (2006). *The laws of simplicity*. Cambridge, MA: MIT Press.

Tufte, E. R. (1990). *Envisioning information*. Cheshire, CT: Graphics Press.

Whitney, D., & Trosten-Bloom, A. (2003). *The power of appreciative inquiry: A practical guide to positive change*. San Francisco: Berrett-Koehler Publishers.

Reflection Questions

1. What is the importance of defining a clear end-point vision prior to implementing a project? What role should stakeholders play in articulating this vision?

2. What role does standards setting play in selecting metrics? Does the role of Donabedian's structure $\rightarrow$ process $\rightarrow$ outcome model play any relevance in choosing metrics?

3. How do the research principles of data validity and reliability tie into data collection in project management? Does data that does not have confirmed validity and reliability play any role in evaluation?

4. How does one determine the cost of data collection and management compared to its relative value in project evaluation?

Learning Activities

1. Take an existing project and determine whether or not clear outcomes for the project were stated early on in the project. Examine who the stakeholders were/should have been to establish these outcomes. Did a data collection plan exist that would measure the impact of the project?

2. Develop measurable and obtainable metrics for a project. Include with these metrics an operational definition to focus on what the metric measures and how it ties to the project. Develop a sampling plan for data collection, including whether the data will be collected in real time or on a retrospective basis. Determine who will collect and display the data and whether it comes from an existing database or must be collected as new data.

3. Prepare a plan for using the data at various phases during and after the project. Anticipate how the data will affect decision making and provide feedback to stakeholders.

References

Austin, C. (1979). *Information systems for hospital administration*. Ann Arbor, MI: Health Administration Press.

Berger, S. (2005). *The power of clinical and financial metrics: Achieving success in your hospital*. Chicago: Health Administration Press.

Carey, R. G., & Lloyd, R. C. (2001). *Measuring quality improvement in healthcare: A guide to statistical process control applications*. Milwaukee, WI: ASQ Quality Press.

Deming, W. E. (1986). *Out of the crisis*. Cambridge, MA: MIT Press.

Fair, D. C. (2004). Statistical process control approaches: Basic theory and use of control charts. In D. E. Lighter & D. C. Fair (Eds.), *Quality management in health care: Principles and methods* (2nd ed., pp. 127–172). Sudbury, MA: Jones and Bartlett.

Fink, A. (1993). *Evaluation fundamentals: Guiding health programs, research, and policy*. Newbury Park, CA: Sage.

Fitzgerald, M. (2004, July 15). Don't stop thinking about the value. *CIO Magazine, 17*(19), 66.

Hayes, B. E. (2008). *Measuring customer satisfaction: Survey design, use, and statistical analysis methods* (3rd ed.). Milwaukee, WI: ASQ Quality Press.

Johantgen, M. (2005). Uses of existing administrative and national databases. In C. Waltz, O. L. Strickland, & E. R. Lenz (Eds.), *Measurement in nursing and health research* (pp. 326–338). New York: Springer.

Kelley, D. L. (1999). *How to use control charts for healthcare*. Milwaukee, WI: ASQ Quality Press.

Lloyd, R. (2004). *Quality health care: A guide to developing and using indicators*. Sudbury, MA: Jones and Bartlett.

Montalvo, I. (2007, September 30). The national database of nursing quality indicators (NDNQI). *OJIN: The Online Journal of Issues in Nursing, 12*(3), Manuscript 2. Retrieved from www.nursingworld.org/MainMenuCategories/ANAMarketplace/ANAperiodicals/OJIN /TableofContents/Volume122007/No3Sept07/NursingQualityIndicators.aspx

Nelson, E. (1995). Report cards or instrument panels: Who needs what? *Journal of Quality Improvement, 21*(4), 155–166.

Ruskin, J. (2010). *The complete works of John Ruskin: Stones of Venice, Volume III*. New York: National Library Association.

Trossman, S. (2006, November–December). Show us the data! NDNQI helps nurses link their care to quality. *The American Nurse, 38*(6), 1, 6.

Whitney, D., & Trosten-Bloom, A. (2003). *The power of appreciative inquiry: A practical guide to positive change*. San Francisco: Berrett-Koehler Publishers.

ELEVEN

Evaluating Project Outcomes

■ Patricia L. Thomas

■ Learning Objectives

1. Discuss data analysis techniques in project management.
2. Describe the importance of outcomes in forecasting future organizational performance.
3. Discuss evaluation methods focusing on *how* and *why* the project works and what is beneath the surface of inputs and outputs.
4. Identify how the project and program plans counter existing causal mechanisms.

> "I learned that courage was not the absence of fear, but the triumph over it. The brave man is not he who does not feel afraid, but he who conquers that fear."
>
> —Nelson Mandela

> "True genius resides in the capacity for evaluation of uncertain, hazardous, and conflicting information."
>
> —Sir Winston Churchill

Key Terms

Casual forecasting

Data-driven decision making

Evidence

Metrics

Performance measures

Qualitative forecasting

Qualitative methods

Simulation forecasting

Time series analysis

Roles

Communicator

Decision maker

Information manager

Integrator

Leader

Risk anticipator

Professional Values

Accountability

Altruism

Integrity

Social justice

Core Competencies

Appreciative inquiry

Assessment

Coordination

Critical thinking

Design

Emotional intelligence

Interpersonal influence

Leadership

Management

Risk reduction

System thinking

Introduction

Evaluating outcomes is central to project management. Often, project evaluation is viewed as a final step in implementation. This is an outdated paradigm as project evaluation starts with design, and the results from the evaluation process often lead to future innovations and revisions in projects. The purpose of this chapter is to examine the evaluation process and propose a new lens to view evaluate methods.

As we consider evaluation and outcomes, it is clear that detailed project plans are the foundation on which meaningful evaluation rests. As practice-focused professionals, we are action oriented and eager to implement change or interventions; however, the planning phase of any project requires more time than is typically allowed. While the value of statistical analysis and data cannot be overstated supporting scholarly activities, the use of qualitative measurement in evaluation is finding its way to evaluation activities as well.

Over the last couple of decades, significant attention has been paid to quality improvement process, strategies, and methods. This has been coupled with establishing an organizational infrastructure to support and inform evaluation. While this infrastructure is important because it represents tools, methods, personnel, and attention to process and measurement or data analysis, alone it proves to be insufficient. As we consider the role of leadership, systems, organizational culture, and evidence-based practices, particularly in sustainability of results, it becomes more evident that evaluation methodology to date has been incomplete.

Berwick (2007), in his keynote address at the Institute for Healthcare Improvement Congress, highlighted the need for practitioners to embrace the softer side of evaluation methods rather than a single-minded focus on randomized clinical trials. This enlightened approach to evaluation brings attention to the context of evaluation grounded in complexity and the nonlinear relationships found in systems. The emphasis is on learning and the need to respect the systems and social situation in which care is provided. Complexity of environments of care and the importance of culture and relationships within organizations is gaining momentum, resonating with members of the nursing profession and practice disciplines. This awareness represents an evolving framework for evaluation and includes both qualitative and quantitative methods.

With general agreement that patient safety needs improvement, it is important for healthcare providers to have a consistent, clear, and concise definition of quality. Lohr (1990) defined quality as ". . . the degree to which health services for individuals and populations increase the likelihood of desired health outcomes and are consistent with current professional knowledge" (p. 4). Systematic, deliberate, and defined methods will be needed to measure, understand, improve, and communicate internal progress at the unit and organization level when programs or projects are identified. This definition of quality becomes the guiding light for project development and evaluation. Organization and practice decisions can then be based on clear measurement, **evidence**, and outcomes supported by a systematic approach to quality and evidence-based practice improvement (Hwang and Herndon, 2007; Newhouse, 2006).

Managing Change: How Do We Evaluate Our Success?

Any project, whether focused on the micro, macro, or mesosystem level, requires an understanding of the readiness for change in the organization. Chapter 1 underscores change and includes technical and contextual understanding of the organization. This is coupled with knowledge of transformational leadership guiding and influencing effective and sustainable change.

From a technical perspective, organizations have invested in educating staff in basic quality and process improvement strategies. This includes problem identification, internal resources for quality and measurement, and committee structures or councils to review and evaluate results. **Metrics** are described as monitors, typically quantitative in nature. Basic skills in identifying sound evidence in the literature and accessing best practices are important components for staff involvement (Huntington et al., 2009; McLaughlin & Kaluzny, 2006; Nelson, Batalden, & Godfrey, 2007).

Considering context and processes of project management, the focus shifts from the *how tos* to elements in the infrastructure, culture, and stakeholder goals to establish what is perceived to be effective, practical, and meaningful to the organization. Concepts of complexity science, change theory, innovation, and implementation science are explored in relation to the project undertaken. Central to contextual understanding of a project is the assessment of leadership support, champion engagement, and the qualitative indicators for success. These are often elusive when benchmarking; executive summaries and interim reports are used to communicate success particularly when organizations primarily devote considerable time and resources to quantitative measurement (McLaughlin & Kaluzny, 2006; Nelson, 2007; Schweikhart & Dembe, 2009). Examples from clinical nurse leaders (CNLs), doctors of nursing practice (DNPs), and executive nurse administrators in this textbook provide sound evidence that engagement of all aspects of project management can be successful.

Scholarship and Its Relationship to Evaluation

Traditionally, scholarship within the profession of nursing focused on dissemination of research and publication of findings in peer-reviewed journals or presentations at professional conferences. Recently, definitions of scholarship within the nursing profession have expanded. The emerging view of scholarship includes the scholarship of discovery and integration; the scholarship of meaning; and the scholarship to resolve practice problems through application of findings (AACN, 2004). The expanded and emerging definitions of scholarship highlight the movement toward translation science and the expectation that scholarship and expanding professional knowledge can and should include application and meaningfulness to practice (AACN, 2004).

An example of this can be found in CNL programs. CNLs are positioned to bring practice changes at the point of care by the provision of evidence-based practice improvement change (AACN, 2007), thus the application of evidence to current practice. Additionally, they are positioned to support systematic review and analysis of complex care concerns identified at the microsystem level amenable to quality improvements that are process and outcome driven. Additional examples can be gleaned from DNP programs. DNP graduates are prepared to evaluate existing evidence and support the creation of new practice evidence to bring about changes in care outcomes. This is based on the understanding and synthesis of research findings, systematic evaluation of current practice, and participation in collaborative research (AACN, 2004; DePalma & McGuire, 2005).

Clearly, DNPs and CNLs are making important contributions by disseminating their work in application, evidence-based practices, linking complex environments of care, and improvement efforts. Examples from their assignments and value-added projects underscore the importance of project management. Consistent and sound evaluations inclusive of quantitative and **qualitative methods** are essential to their contributions for acceptance by members of the healthcare team.

Business Plans: What Is the Connection to Evaluation?

To compete for scarce resources in healthcare organizations, nurses must establish literacy business plan development, articulating support of a proposed program as both fiscally sound and supportive in organizational goal achievement. Business plans encompass quality improvement principles, nursing performance measurement, and the business case for highlighted best practice, workload nursing measures, and the relationship of nursing practices to organizational **performance measures** (Brandt et al., 2009; Montalvo, 2010). As members of a caring discipline, when nurses set out to make change or design a project, the emphasis is often placed on the desire to improve quality, patient safety, or satisfaction. In recent years, inclusion of cost containment, efficiency, and effectiveness have been integrated into planning

(Hwang & Herndon, 2007; Nelson, 2007). A business case provides a concise and descriptive view of a project, highlighting how investment of human and financial resources translates into an economic return that matches or exceeds the original cost or investment when the goals of the project are achieved. To be effective, a business case should address the reasons for a project or change, options, anticipated benefit, costs, and the preferred action steps. Components of a business plan include an executive summary, the service setting, services offered, population served, market analysis for the proposed change, a financial plan, and evidence-based business practices to justify the plan. Each of these components becomes the basis for future program evaluation and considers how the program metrics or measures are used to demonstrate success. Additionally, the business case becomes a framework for championing and marketing the project plans (Brandt et al., 2009).

Regarding quality and patient safety, the business case is predicated on the concepts that a safer healthcare system is more efficient. Using evidence-based practice improvement strategies establishes efficiency and effectiveness, thereby streamlining processes. This provides the organization relevant information that helps to determine if the ultimate goal of a project will be achieved within a framework of cost containment. Drawing connections between concepts allows organizational decision makers to appreciate how a project or program can improve outcomes while contributing to a healthy bottom line (Hwang & Herndon, 2007). Considering this framework, a business case inclusive of analysis of pertinent costs followed by an assessment of options, evidence-based practice improvement strategies would likely have greater opportunity to improve an outcome or achieve a goal.

Errors in treatment, adverse events, and complications are common and costly in the current delivery system (Nelson, 2007). Poor quality care results in more complications and increased costs across the care continuum (Hwang & Herndon, 2007). Making coherent linkages between the costs of these events is part of the business case in establishing long-term improvements. Given the spotlight on care costs, fragmentation of services, and less than desirable outcomes, it is crucial to establish a business case that demonstrates appreciation for the fiscal impact of safety breaches and the case for improved patient safety.

Clinical leaders and experts are expected to address practice concerns within the context of the organization and the culture. The value appropriated to sustaining the improvements is often communicated by indirect means (Montalvo & Dunton, 2007). Additionally, knowledge and skills in quality improvement, data analysis, and evaluation methods, as well as the cultural characteristics of organization are essential to this end. Inclusion of senior leaders articulating the expectation that quality is a shared responsibility for all members of the organization, driven by data, is cornerstone to informing others about the progress of approved programs and projects (Dall, Chen, Seifert, Maddox, & Hogan, 2009).

Improving the quality of care and sustaining these improvements in practice requires several elements. It is important that organizations support a sense of clinical inquiry and questioning so improvement focus areas can be explored. Therefore, leaders must make a commitment to quality improvement grounded in an improvement philosophy and a formal infrastructure supporting principles of measurement and improvement science. Lastly, organizations must be willing to embrace change as the norm enabling transformation of clinical practice.

Forecasting

Irrespective of the business, forecasting concepts are the same. **Forecasting** is a process by which organizations plan for the future. Based on different variables important to a business, forecasting helps predict actions to be taken, establish what outputs are meaningful to the organization, and determine the capacity the organization has to deliver a product or service. Forecasts inform business plans when there is little financial or statistical information available and allow organizations to consider a future state by answering questions about anticipated profit, demand for services or products, costs to produce a product or service, how much money will be required to establish the product or service, a time frame anticipated for return on investment, and consequences if no action is taken (Bushman, 2007).

There are four major categories of forecasting, which are qualitative, time series analysis, causal relationships, and simulation (Chase, Jacobs, & Aquilano, 2005). Qualitative forecasting is subjective and uses estimates and opinions to predict the future. The Delphi method uses surveys in different departments and at various levels of the organization. Each participant responds to surveys or questionnaires with each response being given equal weight or importance in the analysis of the data. Responses to the surveys or questionnaires are compiled and sent back to the participants for further review and revision. The process is repeated until a common forecast consensus is achieved (Chase, Jacobs, & Aquilano, 2005). The Delphi technique is effective in forecasting operations that require coordination across department lines but can be time consuming if significant revisions are needed at each stage of the process. The anonymity of the Delphi method is particularly useful because it engages members throughout the organization, clustered by collective talents, to create a consensus forecast. The forecast is established without interdepartmental fighting that can occur when resources need to be shared. By using the Delphi method, participants do not know the identity of the other participants in the forecasting process and are therefore less likely to generate forecasts that favor one group or aspect of company operations over another.

Another qualitative method is the grass roots method. Grass roots forecasting is based on the assumption that people closest to the customer or the process can predict the business trends of a product or service (Chase et al., 2005). Grass roots forecasting uses a bottom-up approach where those closest to the customer compile their forecasts and submit their information to the next highest level in the organization. The information is revised and passed up to higher levels until it is used as part of the decision-making process in business planning or operations. Grass roots forecasting can have a significant influence on operations if it is used to increase responsiveness to needs that are communicated by the end user. Grass roots forecasting can provide insights into how products are utilized or perceived, establishing both the possibility for market niches and impending market conditions. Having first-hand data can provide insights to enable the tailoring of products and services to meet customer needs and reduce waste (Stanley, 2007).

Time series analysis uses historical data to predict future demands and trends (Chase, Jacobs, & Aquilano, 2005). It uses a series of observations at specified times with a data point at consecutive time periods, which are predetermined and consistent in length. Time series analyses show how performance has changed over time, and predictions about the future are forecasted based on the location of data points that establish the trend line.

Causal forecasting works on the assumption that future results are signaled by a particular variable or indicator. Causal implies the model is attempting to understand the system underlying and surrounding the item being forecasted. This model is limited in scope because the identification of an independent variable must be established as the leading indicator. Causal forecasting includes regression analysis, econometric models, input/output models, and leading indicators (Morneau, 2006). This forecasting method selects a particular statistic, situation, or event to be monitored and then uses the monitored statistic to predict the behavior of another event.

Simulation forecasting allows users to modify different factors and conditions about a particular event or situation to arrive at the prediction of future conditions.

Simulation models use computers to generate a forecast. This type of model is valuable because it allows the user to change costs and volumes to calculate what might happen if the organizational landscape changes.

In concert with a business plan, forecasting outcomes provides a foundation upon which evaluation can be placed. While evidence supports the development and implementation of successful projects and programs, the translation of activities to organizational outcomes is sparse in the literature. When considering the initiatives to improve quality and safety, project selection in an organization is of paramount importance. By establishing a comprehensive business case supported by forecasting, meaningful projects can be conceptualized in support of strategic initiatives and organizational goals. CNLs and DNPs are well positioned to develop the business case and write the business plan. CNLs and DNPs can lead project teams through a disciplined, systematic approach to process analysis, measurement, evaluation of evidence, and evaluation.

Innovative approaches to clinical issues can be frightening as the approach takes the organization outside the traditional or historical boundaries and security of what is known. Using a forecast and business case to structure rationale for new programs serves two purposes. First, it establishes a coherent, thoughtful, and deliberate rationale for members of the organization to consider when making decisions. Second, it provides clear goals, aims, and metrics for measurement to guide evaluation. This is based on a predetermined structure offering equal treatment when considering project approval. Establishing a business plan and forecast facilitates credibility, promoting trust that can be built in the organization through evaluation that demonstrates accuracy of the content provided.

Framework for Quality Improvement and Evidence-Based Practice

As members of a practice discipline, it is imperative that nursing practice be based on science and that guidelines, protocols, and practice standards be reviewed and revised in a systematic manner. Nurses collect data, assess results, participate in quality improvement initiatives, and evaluate outcomes. As such, nurses monitor indicators, collect data, adapt interventions to meet patient needs, and revise protocols. These activities demonstrate that clinical practice is derived from a sense of clinical inquiry that resides in nursing research and evidence-based practice improvement strategies (Hedges, 2006).

The Quality Safety Education for Nurses (QSEN) initiative has challenged the nursing discipline to bring quality improvement and safety into the foreground as an explicit aspect of curricula (QSEN, 2009). Significant changes that include competencies to improve safety and quality of practitioners across disciplines and practice settings have been instituted (Krainovich-Miller, Haber, & Jacobs, 2009; Lachman, Smith-Glasgow, & Donnelly, 2009). A shift in paradigm that recognizes that quality and safety rest in care delivery systems comprised of individual and collective actions within organizations has occurred. Education has shifted away from the sole focus on individuals to emphasize the system. This helps professionals to improve quality and safety in health care by learning how to identify concerns and evaluate, analyze, and improve the healthcare systems in which they practice (Huntington et al., 2009). Using information and learning how to work in interdisciplinary teams underscore the translation of evidence into safe practice.

Irrespective of the quality or process improvement strategy that is embraced by an organization, certain activities are consistent across methodologies. They include a defined aim or purpose; review of the literature; mapping of the current processes; selecting appropriate tools for process analysis; reviewing evidence and best practices, planning for change, and selecting measures and metrics at baseline and for outcomes; and rapid cyclical review of the plan, data, interventions, and outcomes (McLaughlin & Kaluzny, 2006; Nelson, 2007; Newhouse, 2006).

Translation Science

Lachman and colleagues (2009) emphasize that in our current system, it takes 17 years for evidence to translate into practice change. Given the pace of change in healthcare delivery systems, interventions, and technology, a waiting period for the translation of research findings into practice is unacceptable. In the view of Lachman and colleagues, if we rely on evidence-based practices to improve quality, safety, and cost concerns with this track record, it could lead to further fragmentation and collapse of our current system.

Increasing the speed of integration and application of evidence into practice will require both critical and creative thinking. Coupled with attention to organizational support, removing barriers to practice change, and establishing innovative methods for how we educate future practitioners and those currently in practice are crucial (Jones, Mayer, & Mandelkehr, 2009; Lachman et al., 2009; Nelson, 2007).

This requires attention to linear (quantitative) and nonlinear (qualitative) evaluation methods sensitive to systems within organizations.

Data Analysis Techniques in Project Management

No matter what the quality improvement framework or methodology selected by an organization to guide improvement activities, common to all of them is a need to collect data and analyze results. While much has been written about the need for **data-driven decision making**, until recently, data analysis has not been part of the formal curriculum of health professionals.

Data analysis is described in quality improvement, evidence-based practice, research, and project management literature, assuming that individuals have literacy in data analysis. Many pitfalls result from inappropriate inferences drawn from data, yet competency and literacy surrounding data analysis by healthcare professionals is young (Kleinpell, 2009). Many nurses and other health providers have an aversion to data analysis that can, in part, be overcome through education. However, education alone is not sufficient. To develop analytic abilities, practitioners need access to experts in data analysis and management. Decision making has come to rely on data; organizations have invested in the development of data experts who often reside in quality departments. Lean methodology, Six Sigma, and continuous improvement rely on measurement and statistical methods to support reporting functions (McLaughlin & Kaluzny, 2006; Shulman, 2008).

If your organization does not have data experts, consultants and statisticians can be engaged to support projects. Engage the help of your data manager or statistician during the design phase of the project to ensure appropriate data elements are identified for measurement metrics.

Benchmarks and Report Cards

In recent years, the practice of measuring and reporting performance of health systems and processes has increased. Organizations throughout the country are now required to publish outcomes and metrics to comply with contractual and regulatory obligations at the local, state, and national levels. By comparing the performance of providers and organizations with established and defined metrics, better performance is encouraged.

While public reporting of quality indicators can be used to identify areas for improvement, many organizations are turning to benchmarking performance within their health system and with comparable competitors to establish strengths and proactively identify areas needing improvement (Hughes, 2008).

Benchmarking in health care is defined as a disciplined and systematic application of continuous measures of defined indicators for the purpose of comparison to others. Benchmarking allows organizations to evaluate the results of key processes that have distinct and consistent definitions. Benchmarking for the purposes of improving patient safety and quality can be done as an internal comparison of metrics or measurement between comparable units within an organization or as an external process in which an organization compares itself to like organizations in the state or country (Hughes, 2008).

Internal benchmarking is used to identify best practices within the organization, to compare best practices within an organization, or to compare current practice over time. Information and data are plotted on a control chart for trending purposes, allowing the organization to establish the consistency of the process embedded in the defined metric over time. A limit of internal benchmarking is that an organization's current practice may not represent best practices elsewhere (Hughes, 2008).

External benchmarking involves using comparative data between organizations to evaluate performance and identify improvements that have proven to be successful in other organizations. Comparative national data is available from the Agency for Healthcare Research and Quality, the Centers for Medicare and Medicaid Services, and proprietary benchmarking groups such as the American Nurses Association's National Database of Nursing Quality Indicators (Hughes, 2008).

Dodek, Heyland, Rocker, and Cook (2004) identified that report cards or instrument panels have become a popular way to present performance data. Report cards are summative evaluations of clinical outcomes that reflect past practice and can be used to display internal or external comparison benchmarks. Report cards provide a visual depiction of performance, often used to assist consumers and providers in decision making pertaining to where they want to receive care. Instrument panels are formative evaluations of processes, outcomes, or cost that reflect a snapshot in time of the current performance. A combination of summative and formative evaluation is called the balanced scorecard.

Evaluation of projects is multifaceted, built from quantitative and qualitative methods that embrace research, evidence, and systems thinking. Our current healthcare delivery systems recognize that elevating clinical practice, improvement outcomes, and addressing concerns in quality and safety will require an approach that includes deliberate and systematic evaluation inclusive of measurement and an understanding of the context and impact the change has on the participant systems. DNPs are uniquely prepared and positioned to bridge the gap between where we are and where we want to be. Recognizing no single ingredient is sufficient to bring effective evaluation to every situation, the blend of quantitative and qualitative methods, review of evidence and best practices, consideration of research findings, and thoughtful, systematic synthesis will provide meaningful evaluation to improve outcomes.

Summary

- Meaningful project evaluation begins with a detailed business case and project plan that includes critical indicators and expected outcomes.
- Evaluation of change, programs, and projects includes qualitative and quantitative measures.
- Irrespective of the quality philosophy employed in an organization, improvement relies on a systematic and disciplined approach to understanding and evaluating process.
- Evidence-based practices inform the selection of appropriate interventions to support quality care and data-driven outcomes.

Suggested Readings

Bennett, L., & Slavin, L. (2002). *Continuous quality improvement: What every health care manager needs to know.* Retrieved from http://www.case.edu/med/epidbio/mphp439/CQI.htm

Committee on Quality of Health Care in America, Institute of Medicine. (1999). *To err is human: Building a safer health system.* Washington, DC: National Academies Press.

Committee on Quality of Health Care in America, Institute of Medicine. (2001). *Crossing the quality chasm: A new health system for the 21st century.* Washington, DC: National Academies Press.

Cronenwett, L., Sherwood, G., Barnsteiner, J., Disch, J., Johnson, J., Mitchell, P., et al. (2007). Quality and safety education for nurses. *Nursing Outlook, 55*(3), 122–131.

Hughes, R. (2008). Tools and strategies for quality improvement and patient safety. In *Patient safety and quality: An evidence-based handbook for nurses* (Ch. 44). Agency for Healthcare Research and Quality, Publication No. 08-0043. Retrieved from http://www.ahrq.gov/qual /nurseshdbk/docs/HughesR_QMBMP.pdf

The Joint Commission. (2008). *Health care at the crossroads: Guiding principles for the development of the hospital of the future.* Retrieved from http://www.jointcommission.org /NR/rdonlyres/1C9A7079-7A29-4658-B80D-A7DF8771309B/0/Hosptal_Future.pdf

Newhouse, R., Pettit, J., Poe, S, & Rocco, L. (2006). The slippery slope: Differentiating between quality improvement and research. *Journal of Nursing Administration, 36*(4), 211–219.

Reinhardt, A., & Ray, L. (2003). Differentiating quality improvement from research. *Applied Nursing Research, 15*, 2–8.

Reflection Questions

1. In terms of project evaluation, for what methods do you feel most prepared? For what do you feel least prepared?
2. What resources are available in your organization to assist you with project evaluation, data management, analysis, and dissemination?
3. How do you see the DNP or CNL interacting with members of the healthcare team to advance quality improvement, evidence-based practices, and evaluation?

Learning Activities

1. Interview a DNP or CNL within your organization to identify the methods, tools, and measurement techniques typically employed. Can you identify areas to expand?
2. Outline the steps you would undertake to organize a clinical improvement project. What methods would you use to evaluate your progress and effectiveness for each of the activities?
3. Examine a project that used traditional, quantitative methods for evaluation. Identify qualitative methods that could be used to add value to the findings.

Role Descriptions for DNPs and CNLs

AACN Position Statement on the Practice Doctorate in Nursing: http://www .aacn.nche.edu/DNP/DNPPositionStatement.htm

AACN *White Paper on the Role of the Clinical Nurse Leader:* http://www .aacn.nche.edu/Publications/WhitePapers/ClinicalNurseLeader07.pdf

The Essentials of Doctoral Education for Advanced Nursing Practice: http://www.aacn.nche.edu/DNP/pdf/Essentials.pdf

Resources

Agency for Health Care Research and Quality: http://www.ahrq.gov

Centers for Medicare and Medicaid Services: www.cms.hhs.gov

Cochrane Collaboration: http://www.cochrane.org

Institute for Healthcare Improvement: http://www.ihi.org

Joanna Briggs Institute: http://www.joannabriggs.edu.au

The Joint Commission: www.jointcommission.org

National Quality Forum: www.qualityforum.org

Time Series Analysis: http://www.itl.nist.gov/div898/handbook/pmc/section4/pmc4.htm

References

American Association of Colleges of Nursing. (2004). *Doctor of nursing practice roadmap taskforce report.* Retrieved from http://www.aacn.nche.edu/dnp/pdf/DNP.pdf

American Association of Colleges of Nursing. (2007). *White paper on the education and role of the clinical nurse leader.* Retrieved from http://www.aacn.nche.edu/Publications/WhitePapers/2-07.pdf

Berwick, D. (2007). Eating soup with a fork. *IHI Congress.* Retrieved from http://www.ihi.org/IHI/Programs/AudioAndWebPrograms/OnDemandPresentationBerwick.htm

Brandt, J., Edwards, D., Sullivan, S., Zehler, J., Grinder, S., Scott, K., et al. (2009). An evidence-based business planning process. *Journal of Nursing Administration, 39*(12), 511–513.

Bushman, M. (2007). *Why is forecasting important to an organization?* Retrieved from http://www.associatedcontent.com/article/200360/why_is_forecasting_important_to_an.html?cat=3

Chase, R., Jacobs, F., & Aquilano, N. (2005). *Operations management for competitive advantage* (11th ed.). New York: McGraw-Hill.

Dall, T., Chen Y., Seifert R., Maddox P., & Hogan, P. (2009). The economic value of professional nursing. *Med Care, 47,* 97–104.

DePalma, J., & McGuire, P. (2010). *Course description at Purdue University,* Indianapolis, IN.

Dodek, P., Heyland, D., Rocker, G., & Cook, D. (2004). Translating family satisfaction data into quality improvement. *Critical Care Medicine, 32*(9), 1922–1927.

Dunton, N., & Montalvo, I. (2009). *Sustained improvement in nursing quality: Hospital performance on NDNQI indicators 2007–2008.* Silver Spring, MD: American Nurses Association.

Hedges, C. (2006). Research, evidence-based practice, and quality improvement: The 3-legged stool. *AACN Advanced Critical Care, 17*(4), 457–459.

Hughes, R. (2008). Tools and strategies for quality improvement and patient safety. In *Patient safety and quality: An evidence-based handbook for nurses* (Ch. 44). Agency for Healthcare Research and Quality, Publication No. 08-0043, Retrieved from http://www.ahrq.gov/qual /nurseshdbk/docs/HughesR_QMBMP.pdf

Huntington, J., Dycus, P., Hix, C., West, R., McKeon, L., Coleman, M., et al. (2009). A standardized curriculum to introduce novice health professional students to practice-based learning and improvement: A multi-institutional pilot study. *Quality Management in Health Care, 18*(3), 174–181.

Hwang, R., & Herndon, J. (2007). The business case for patient safety. *Clinical Orthopaedics and Related Research, 457,* 21–34.

Jones, C., Mayer, C., & Mandelkehr, L. (2009). Innovations at the intersection of academia and practice: Facilitating graduate nursing students' learning about quality improvement and patient safety. *Quality Management in Healthcare, 18*(3), 158–164.

Kleinpell, R. (2009). Promoting research in clinical practice: Strategies for implementing research initiatives. *Journal of Trauma Nursing, 16*(2), 114–119.

Krainovich-Miller, B., Haber, J., & Jacobs, S. (2009). Evidence-based practice challenge: Teaching critical appraisal of systematic reviews and clinical practice guidelines to graduate students. *Journal of Nursing Education, 48*(4), 186–195.

Lachman, V., Smith-Glasgow, M., & Donnelly, G. (2009). Teaching innovation, *Nursing Administration Quarterly, 33*(3), 205–211.

Lohr, K. (1990). *Medicare: A strategy for quality assurance.* Washington, DC: National Academy Press.

McLaughlin, C. P., & Kaluzny, A. D. (2006). *Continuous quality improvement in health care: Theory, implementation, and applications* (3rd ed.). Sudbury, MA: Jones and Bartlett.

Montalvo, I. (2010). Developing a quality landscape. *Men in Nursing, 40*(1), 10–12.

Montalvo, I., & Dunton, N. (2007). *Transforming nursing data into quality care: Profiles of quality improvement in U.S. healthcare facilities.* Silver Spring, MD: American Nurses Association.

Morneau, M. (2006). *Forecasting models.* Retrieved from http://www.associatedcontent.com /article/62649/forecasting_models.html?cat=6

Nelson, E., Batalden, P., & Godfrey, M. (2007). *Quality by design. A clinical microsystems approach.* San Francisco: Jossey-Bass.

Newhouse, R. (2006). Selecting measures for safety and quality improvement initiatives, *Journal of Nursing Administration, 36*(3), 109–113.

Newhouse, R. (2007). Diffusing confusion among evidence-based practice, quality improvement, and research. *Journal of Nursing Administration, 37*(10), 432–435.

Quality and Safety Education for Nurses. (2010). Accessed on May 12, 2010, at http://www
.qsen.org

Schweikhart, S., & Dembe, A. (2009). The applicability of lean and Six Sigma techniques to
clinical and translational research, *Journal of Investigative Medicine, 57*(7), 748–755.

Shulman, C. (2008). Strategies for starting a successful evidence-based practice program. *Advanced
Critical Care, 19*(3), 301–311.

Stanley, O. (2007). *Forecasting methods for business to business success.* Retrieved from http://
www.associatedcontent.com/article/273323/forecasting_methods_for_business_to_pg4
.html?cat=4

TWELVE

Disseminating Results as a Mechanism for Sustaining Innovation

■ Anna C. Alt-White and Maryann F. Pranulis

■ **Learning Objectives**

1. Determine the best mechanisms for communicating project outcomes.
2. Identify essential elements to manage and share information.
3. Describe characteristics of professional presentations.

> "Knowing is not enough; we must apply.
>
> Willing is not enough; we must do."
>
> —Goethe

Key Terms

Appreciative inquiry
Mind mapping
Social networking

Storytelling
Sustainability
Variability

Roles

Communicator
Decision maker
Information manager

Integrator
Leader
Risk anticipator

Professional Values

Communality of knowledge
Inquisitiveness
Integrity

Objectivity
Social justice

Core Competencies

Assessment
Critical thinking
Emotional intelligence

Interpersonal influence
Risk taking
Systems approach

Introduction

Creating a Lasting Impression

Some efforts are like footsteps in the sand that last only until the next wave hits the shore. Other efforts are cast in concrete, never to be erased (unless blown apart) and live long beyond their usefulness or intended purpose. Use of contemporary, **appreciative inquiry** methods and systems thinking achieves a happy medium and provides a mechanism for achieving endurance (i.e., sustainability) in the face of change (Havens, Wood, & Leeman, 2006; Marchionni & Richer, 2007). An ancient Chinese proverb provides insight into the mechanism that enables both endurance and adaptability. "Give a man a fish, and he eats for a day. Teach him how to fish, and he eats for a lifetime." This chapter promotes sustainability of innovations, tempered with adaptability. It aims to provide recommendations for teaching the audience for dissemination of information about how to "fish" rather than teaching them how to replicate an innovation in its entirety.

Using the Purpose, Audience, Presentation, Evidence, and Language Model

There are five basic components of any presentation of information. They include purpose, audience, presentation, evidence, and language (PAPEL) (Miller, 1992). **Table 12-1** provides definitions of these terms. In the PAPEL model, the term *presentation* encompasses the full range of oral, written, and technical means of disseminating information. The interaction between and among these components creates the positive, neutral, or negative synergy of a presentation and the audience's subsequent motivation to adopt or adapt the innovation in their settings. To ensure the presentation has a positive impact, it is important that the innovation-specific presentation components are well thought out and planned to be appropriately complementary and harmonious. The greater the knowledge and understanding of the PAPEL components for a particular presentation, the greater the ability to produce a scholarly presentation having a substantial effect. Reference to the PAPEL model components is made throughout this chapter to illustrate their application in different situations.

Table 12-1 PAPEL Model for Developing Dynamite Presentations

Component	Definition
Purpose	Explicit: Stated reason for presentation
	Implicit: What you actually hope to accomplish
Audience	Intended: Persons you are aiming to reach
	Actual: Persons who are exposed to the presentation
Presentation	Mode of presenting information: Oral or written; with or without audiovisual aids; spontaneous or planned; formal or informal

(continues)

Table 12-1 PAPEL Model for Developing Dynamite Presentations *(continued)*

Component	Definition
Evidence	Content: Information being conveyed and supported by data, facts, opinion, direct observation, reference to the work of others, hearsay
Language	Level of diction and formality: Voice and tense; objectivity vs. self-reference; scientific/professional vs. lay terminology or street language

Organization of the Chapter

It is essential to know one's own skills and limitations and use them deliberately to enhance the presentation. Using the system's approach and appreciative inquiry methods provides opportunities to capitalize on the skills and talents of various members of the innovation team as well as the leader. To better understand this approach, appreciative inquiry is defined:

> Appreciative Inquiry (AI) is about the coevolutionary search for the best in people, their organizations, and the relevant world around them. In its broadest focus, it involves systematic discovery of what gives "life" to a living system when it is most alive, most effective, and most constructively capable in economic, ecological, and human terms. AI involves, in a central way, the art and practice of asking questions that strengthen a system's capacity to apprehend, anticipate, and heighten positive potential. (Cooperrider & Whitney, 2010, p.1).

Appreciative inquiry provides the context for disseminating results as a mechanism for sustaining innovation. Therefore, the chapter begins with a discussion of personal style followed by continuous assessment of the innovation and the available resources as they are located in the space–time continuum. The chapter concludes with a discussion of differences and similarities of formal professional and informal presentations.

Personal Style

Everyone has unique strengths and characteristics that mesh well with different people and situations at different times. Identifying and capitalizing on these strengths and matching them with audience characteristics early in the innovation process are keys to making successful presentations to different audiences. Presentation of information about an innovation is successful if it is remembered favorably and implemented or applied to new situations.

Personal style includes physical appearance, ease of interacting in different settings, vocal qualities—including volume, tone, pitch, and intonations and personal power. Habitual and deliberate use of gestures, ease of making eye contact, ability to listen, ability to communicate interest in and enthusiasm about the topic, and willingness to accept criticism can add or detract from a presentation. Awareness of personal styles of each member of the innovation team allows flexibility in matching personal style to situation and audience needs (Rutledge, Bajaj, & Mucciolo, 2007).

In the traditional sense, a project and its outcomes are usually not communicated until completion. Conversely, an innovation is not considered complete until its outcomes are disseminated. Within the appreciative inquiry framework, dissemination of information takes place throughout the process of innovation. This is an essential component of creating transparency for an evidence-based practice culture (Marchionni & Richer, 2007). The approach to be used for disseminating information throughout the project requires forethought, leadership flexibility, willingness to capitalize on the presentation strengths of the team members, and the ability to view the innovation process in its entirety.

Looking at the Whole Picture

Sustainability of an innovation or its "stickiness" requires an understanding of the factors impacting dissemination, adoption, and sustainability of innovations (Havens et al., 2006). Olivia and Rockart (1997) identified resources that are needed to sustain an innovation.

1. Employee time
2. Managerial time
3. Project and program tools

Employee time must be balanced with the project and throughout the activities that are associated with implementation and projected outcomes. Insufficient manager time can constrain growth for a project or program, thus becoming a barrier to sustainment. If employees and managers lack the skill sets for planning, activating, and evaluating outcomes, project and program life cycles are short. For long-term clinical program sustainability that allows systems to brand outcomes and disseminate knowledge, a capital plan that includes the following three components is needed.

1. Ongoing operating costs
2. Maintenance of the project/program equipment
3. Capital equipment depreciation and replacement (Health Canada, 2010)

Because dissemination entails an ongoing exchange of information between and among the project leader and the staff (King, Hawe, & Wise, 1998), planning for dissemination starts at the same time the project is being developed (Pluye, Potvin, Denis, Pelletier, & Mannoni, 2005; Southwell, Gannaway, Orrell, Chalmers, & Abraham, 2005). As stated by Green, Ottoson, Garcia, and Hiatt (2009), "Dissemination is not an end in itself; its intended benefits depend on integration and implementation by the end users, who will also determine the relevance and usability of whatever is disseminated" (p 168).

Scheirer's (2005) systematic review identified five factors influencing program sustainability, which include modification of the program, having a champion, fit with the organization's mission and procedures, perceived benefits to staff and/or clients, and support from stakeholders in other organizations (Brownson, Kreuter, Arrington, & True, 2006; Greenhalgh, Robert, MacFarlane, Bate, & Kyriakidou, 2004; Rogers, 2003; Scheirer, 2005). **Table 12-2** presents a list of some of the factors and conditions that influence dissemination, adoption, and sustainability.

Table 12-2 Influences on Dissemination, Adoption, and Sustainability of Innovations

Influences	Optimal Condition
Relative advantage	More advantageous than alternatives
Compatibility	Consistent with values, past experiences, and needs
Complexity	Easy to understand and use
Trialability	Easy to implement on a limited basis
Observability	Results visible
Risk	Balance between risks and benefits
Reversibility	Ability to reinstate previous approach if innovation doesn't work

Table 12-2 Influences on Dissemination, Adoption, and Sustainability of Innovations
(continued)

Influences	Optimal Condition
Cost	Benefits outweigh the costs
Revisability	Easy to adapt
Reinvention	Ability to adapt, refine, or modify innovation to meet needs
Knowledge	Easy to codify and transfer from one context to another
Augmentation support	Provides support, e.g., help desk, training
Task issues	Relevant and improves work performance
Leadership	Shared vision; clear goals; stability and consistency; committed; recognition and reward of participants
Readiness for change	Recognizing need to change; dynamic policy systems
Resources	Availability of funds, expertise, time, development, and training
Communication	Information flow, e.g., technology and face-to-face discussion

Sustainability of a project and programs is often influenced by costs and **variability**, especially in clinical settings. Cost as an influencing factor centers around three common areas.

1. Cost benefit (cost and benefits valued in cash terms)
2. Cost effectiveness (outcomes measured in natural units; symptom reduction, years of life gained)
3. Cost utility (outcomes measured in a composite of both length and quality of life)

Creating value chains that link to quality outcomes yields sustainable projects and cost containment. However, costs can spiral out of control and projects/programs will not be sustained if variability is not considered as a real or anticipated barrier or influence. Variability can be nonrandom and unnecessary, but controllable.

For example, scheduling discharges is a way to control variability. High variability leads to peaks and troughs in resource demands and stresses systems. Artificial peaks cause delays and diversion for programs and clinical programs regardless of how well results are communicated and disseminated in the organization.

One strategy to consider for managing variability is queuing theory. The method focuses on supply, demand, service, utilization, intensity, and probability associated with services and requests (Gorunesau, McClean, & Millard, 2002; Gross & Harris, 1998). Another example is the application of lean theory where value is added, waste is removed, and flow is enhanced. Thus, variability is reduced and the potential for project and program **sustainability** is increased (McManus, Long, Cooper, & Litvak, 2004).

Fitting the Pieces Into the Whole

At any time that a presentation is made about the innovation or the project, it is essential to bring the audience into the context of the situation; the innovation should be made pertinent to their interests and needs. It is advisable to inform the audience about the situation giving rise to the innovation (the *why*) as well as the nature of the innovation (the *what*) and who is/was involved. To make the presentation interesting to the audience (both intended and actual), the members of the audience need to understand how they affect or are affected by both the process and product of the innovation.

It is tempting to focus solely on describing the innovation. But meaning is derived only in context. Therefore, it helps to point out how the innovation fits the system's structure and function as well as the specific audience's needs and interests. This includes, for an executive decision-making audience, discussing how the innovation fits the organization's mission and goals, and the cost impact in terms of financial, human, technical, and other resources. For a unit-based presentation, a more useful discussion includes quality-of-care issues, how the innovation impacts individual and unit efficiency and effectiveness, and how it will benefit the patient, the staff, and the staff's relationships with other components of the organization.

Regardless of the level of formality of the presentation, the content must be presented in a logical sequence. The logic can be based on a standard format of problem, analysis, intervention, results, and discussion, or it can be based on a logical flow of ideas, a chronologic sequence of events, or some other logical schematic that helps the audience follow the content of the presentation. Outlines, summaries of the presentation, tables, conceptual diagrams, **mind mapping**, fishbone diagrams, flow charts, and other visual aids help to demonstrate the logic underlying both the presentation and the innovation. Prepared and spontaneous illustrations using whiteboards, bulletin boards, or computer-generated diagrams help to show how the innovation (the piece) fits into the system as a whole.

This Is a Process, Not a Product

Innovation is a process. Communication about and throughout the process evokes a sense of transparency and interest in the project or program and eventually garners support and sustainability. The evidence (research data, facts, literature, cost and/or quality data, and observations) that is used will vary in keeping with both the stage of the process and the audience. During the planning stage, it is appropriate to use (as evidence to support the need) published reports, publicly available data sets, or quality improvement reports. For the implementation phase, desirable evidence consists of summations of ongoing records, minutes, journals, general note taking and even photographs that best describe the status of the project. The documentation then becomes the source for generating interim reports. Upon achievement of the initial and final goals, formal and informal presentations are made relying on the process and outcomes data generated throughout the innovation.

Timing Is Crucial

The following three aspects of timing affect the success and sustainability of an innovation: relevance of topic, strategic planning with timelines, and room for changes and unexpected events. An innovation can be brilliant and executed to perfection. But if the timing is not congruent with environmental conditions (e.g., organizational needs and events in the larger community and world), it will not be relevant to the times. It may be considered premature or after the fact and not needed. Unless viewed as needed, the innovation may not be implementable or sustained if implemented.

Managing the project calls for committing to a strategic plan (timelines and milestones) that includes periodic and terminal reports. The reports can be viewed as subprojects and, like the overall plan, should have time included for planning, preparation, and execution of the presentation. Regular internal meetings and external professional meetings should be noted in the strategic plan because they provide opportunities to disseminate information. All of the timelines (including presentations) need to incorporate time for delays, unexpected events, and starting over or redrafting—time for changes and unexpected events.

Characteristics of Professional Presentations

There are countless tools for disseminating information about innovations. The major categories are **social networking**, written reports, presentations, and news media (see **Table 12-3**). The suggested readings for this chapter provide detailed information about using these tools. A key resource is Rutledge and colleagues' (2007) *Special Edition: Using Microsoft Office PowerPoint 2007*. This reference explains how to prepare PowerPoint presentations. In addition, they include extensive information about presentation design (i.e., scripting the concept, designing visual support and selecting the best medium for the message), presentation skills, and presenting in a variety of settings. Other suggested readings describe in detail how to prepare visual aids (i.e., tables, posters, bulletin boards, or websites) and steps for submitting manuscripts to professional journals.

Table 12-3   Tools for Disseminating Information About Innovations

Media for Message	Tools	Cautions
Social networking	■ Appreciative inquiry ■ Informal face-to-face communication ■ E-mail ■ Wikis ■ Web log (blogging, e.g., Facebook, Twitter, MySpace)	■ Interpersonal/group dynamics ■ Loss of confidentiality ■ No exclusive owner of content ■ Headline approach; lacks details ■ "Tell one person, you tell the world"; no control over dissemination of original message

Table 12-3   Tools for Disseminating Information About Innovations *(continued)*

Media for Message	Tools	Cautions
Written reports	■ Business case ■ Internal project reports—interim and final ■ Reports to external regulating bodies ■ Journal articles	■ Avoid verbosity and redundancy ■ Adherence to guidelines for type of report
Presentations	■ PowerPoint presentations ■ Flip charts/overheads ■ Storyboards ■ Slides ■ Videos ■ Posters ■ Handouts	■ Equipment failure ■ Cumbersome ■ May get lost in transit; make backups
News media	Press releases and interviews for: ■ Television ■ Radio ■ Newspapers ■ Magazines	■ May or may not be quoted or published verbatim; try to get authorization to do final review/approval ■ Selective audience

An innovator must be a salesperson who persuades others to see the value of the project. Communication is critical and "good presentation skills work everywhere" (Rutledge et al., 2007, p. 559). Modifying how the information is presented and structured can affect the extent of the impact (Gladwell, 2002). Presentation format, content, supporting evidence, and even presenter attire will vary depending on the audience. For example, a formal presentation to the board of directors of a large healthcare system may require using a specified format for a written report that will be submitted in advance of the meeting. At the time of the in-person presentation, the presenter wears business attire, uses business language to support professional/scientific terminology, and emphasizes cost savings and improving care. Staying within the time allotted is crucial.

In contrast, a presentation to the nursing staff on an involved unit in a healthcare system will be less formal and more interactive. Generally, the presenter wears normal work attire. The presentation may include using a PowerPoint slide show, a whiteboard, a bulletin board, or posters to illustrate points. It is helpful to distribute written information in advance of or at the meeting. In place of a full written report, a one-page summary or outline may be more useful. Here the emphasis is on improving care and the value to the patient and the staff. Like more formal presentations, it is important to be organized and concise and to stay within the allotted time.

A podium presentation to a scientific or professional audience will follow a specified format, use audiovisual aids, and will emphasize data and facts presented objectively followed by interpretation of the data that may include self-reference. Scientific and professional terminology is used and the presenter wears professional attire. The presenter is usually physically distant from the audience in a darkened room, which makes it difficult to read and adjust to the audience. A poster presentation at the same meeting also uses audiovisual aids, but they are displayed for a longer period of time and there is opportunity for dialogue with the audience. Poster presentations using slides similar to those in a PowerPoint presentation can also be a scholarly way of sharing project results. This gives the authors the opportunity to give details of their process, identifying barriers overcome and lessons learned along the way.

In contrast, a presentation to a lay audience composed of adolescents should also be fact based, but rely on a **storytelling** approach peppered with self-reference (i.e., how the presenter became interested in or worked on the innovation). To reach the audience the presenter may wear casual rather than business attire and use lay terminology and even street language interspersed with the appropriate professional terms.

Press releases to newspapers, newsletters, websites, radio, and television are important means for informing both specific and general audiences. They should be brief and address the five Ws and H of journalism—who? what? when? where? why? and how? Content for written releases are easier to control, and most organizations have a public relations department that will either generate the release, assist with developing it, and/or clear it for release. However, there is no guarantee that the information—when in print or in the news—will match the written, authentic press release. It is much more difficult to control what is included in interviews. Although it is not appropriate to read from a script for an interview, it is helpful to have the key points on note cards and to provide the interviewer with a written copy of the correct information.

Summary

- Dissemination of information about an innovation is crucial to its approval, acceptance, and sustainability.
- Use of the PAPEL model facilitates planning the timing, approach, content, and success of a presentation.
- The appointed leader of an innovation effort may or may not be the appropriate person to make audience-specific presentations.
- Functioning within the appreciative inquiry philosophy and mode encourages using the talents and skills of the innovation team to their best advantage throughout the innovation effort.
- Continuous communication and dissemination of information promotes transparency and time for doing, and so they should be included in the strategic plan.
- A measure of success for dissemination of innovation information is audience interest in approving, implementing, and sustaining the innovation.

Suggested Readings

The subject matter addressed follows each suggested reading in parentheses.

Ambler, M. (2009, January). Social media and the health care leader: Maximizing your information intake. *Voice of Nursing Leadership,* 10–12. (Social networking)

Barnett, L. M., Van Beurden, E., Eakin, E. G., Beard, J., Dietrich, U., & Newman, B. (2004). Program sustainability of a community-based intervention to prevent falls among older Australians. *Health Promotion International, 19*(3), 281–288. doi:10.1093/heapro/dah302 (Sustainability)

Evans, M. L. (2000). Polished, professional presentation: Unlocking the design elements. *The Journal of Continuing Education in Nursing, 31*(5), 213–218. (Presentation basics)

Happell, B. (2005). Disseminating nursing knowledge—A guide to writing for publication. *The International Journal of Psychiatric Nursing Research, 10*(3), 1147–1155. (Publication preparation)

Hess, G. R., Tosney, K. W., & Liegel, L. H. (2009). Creating effective poster presentations: AMEE guide no. 40. *Medical Teacher, 31,* 319–321. doi:10/1080/01421690902826131 (Poster presentations)

LaPelle, N. R., Zapka, J., & Ockene, J. K. (2006). Sustainability of public health programs: The example of tobacco treatment services in Massachusetts. *American Journal of Public Health, 96*(8), 1363–1369. doi:10.2105/AJPH.2005.067124 (Sustainability)

Robinson, K., Elliott, S. J., Driedger, M., Eyles, J., O'Loughlin, J., Riley, B., et al. (2005). Using linking systems to build capacity and enhance dissemination in heart health promotion: A

Canadian multiple-case study. *Health Education Research, 20*(5), 499–513. doi:10.1093
/her/cyh006 (Dissemination)

Rutledge, P. A., Bajaj, G., & Mucciolo, T. (2007). *Special edition: Using Microsoft Office
PowerPoint ® 2007.* Indianapolis, IN: QUE. (All forms of presentations)

Stetler, C. B., McQueen, L., Demakis, J., & Mittman, B. S. (2008). An organizational framework
and strategic implementation for system-level change to enhance research-based practice:
QUERI series. *Implementation Science, 3*(30), http://www.implementationscience.com
/content/3/1/30. doi:10.1186/1748-5908-3-30 (Implementation of change)

Reflection Question

Identify who is involved in the problem being corrected, who is involved in planning
and implementing the innovation, who is affected by the innovation or its outcomes,
and who are the decision makers. Identify what will be communicated, in what
manner, to each of these groups.

Learning Activities

1. For a month, do stream-of-consciousness journal writing.
2. Prepare an audiovisual presentation tailored to two contrasting audiences.

References

Brownson, R. C., Kreuter, M. W., Arrington, B. A., & True, W. R. (2006). Translating scientific
discoveries into public health action: How can schools of public health move us forward?
Public Health Reports, 121, 97–103.

Cooperrider, D., & Whitney, D. (2010). *A positive revolution in change: Appreciative inquiry.*
[Excerpt]. Retrieved from http://appreciativeinquiry.case.edu/intro/whatisai.cfm

Gladwell, M. (2002). *The tipping point: How little things can make a big difference.* New York:
Little, Brown & Co.

Gorunescu, F., McClean, S. L., & Millard, P. J. (2002). Using queueing model to help plan bed
allocation in the department of geriatric medicine. *Health Care Management Science, 5*(4),
307–312.

Green, L. W., Ottoson, J. M., Garcia, C., & Hiatt, R. A. (2009). Diffusion theory and knowledge
dissemination, utilization, and integration in public health. *Annual Review of Public Health,
30*, 151–174. doi:10.1146/annurev.publhealth.031308.100049

Greenhalgh, T., Robert, G., MacFarlane, F., Bate, P., & Kyriakidou, O. (2004). Diffusion of
innovations in service organizations: Systematic review and recommendations. *The Milbank
Quarterly, 82*(4), 581–629.

Gross, D., & Harris, C. M. (1998). *Fundamentals of queueing theory* (3rd ed). Indianapolis, IN: Wiley & Sons.

Havens, D. S., Wood, S. O., & Leeman, J. (2006). Improving nursing practice and patient care: Building capacity with appreciative inquiry. *JONA: The Journal of Nursing Administration, 36*(10), 463–470.

Health Canada, First Nations, Inuit, and Aboriginal Health. (2010). *Sustainability, reporting and monitoring activities.* Retrieved from http://www.hc-sc.gc.ca/fniah-spnia/pubs/services/_home-domicile/handbook-guide_3b/3b_3_sustain-viable-eng.php

King, L., Hawe, P., & Wise, M. (1998). Making dissemination a two-way process. *Health Promotion International, 13*(3), 237–244.

Marchionni, C., & Richer, M. C. (2007). Using appreciative inquiry to promote evidence-based practice in nursing: The glass is more than half full. *Nursing Leadership, 20*(3), 86–97.

McManus, M. L., Long, M. C., Cooper, A., & Litvak, E. (2004). Queuing theory accurately models the need for critical resources. *Anesthesiology, 100*(5), 1271–1276.

Miller, S. (1992). Writing emphasis course. *Personal communication.* University of Utah.

Olivia, R., & Rockart, S. (1997). Dynamics of multiple improvement efforts: The program life cycle model. Retrieved from http://www.systemdynamics.org/conferences/1997/paper166.htm

Pluye, P., Potvin, L., Denis, J. L., Pelletier, J., & Mannoni, C. (2005). Program sustainability begins with the first events. *Evaluation and Program Planning, 28*(2), 123–137. doi:10.1016/j.evalprogplan.2004.10.003

Rogers, E. M. (2003). *Diffusion of innovations* (5th ed.). New York: Free Press.

Rutledge, P. A., Bajaj, G., & Mucciolo, T. (2007). *Special edition: Using Microsoft Office PowerPoint ® 2007.* Indianapolis, IN: QUE.

Scheirer, M. A. (2005). Is sustainability possible? A review and commentary on empirical studies of program sustainability. *American Journal of Evaluation, 26*(3), 320–347. doi:10.1177/1098214005278752

Southwell, D., Gannaway, D., Orrell, J., Chalmers, D., & Abraham, C. (2005). *Strategies for effective dissemination of project outcomes.* Commonwealth of Australia: University of Queensland and Flinders University. Retrieved from http://hdl.handle.net/10096/217

THIRTEEN

Voices From the Field

Executive Nurse Administration, Clinical Nurse Leader, and Doctor of Nursing Practice Student Assignment Examples, Information From Professors, and Student Exemplars

■ **Linda Roussel, Catherine Dearman, and Lonnie K. Williams**

■ **Learning Objective**

Identify components of student project assignments and examples that support project and program sustainability.

> **"What you do not know, you can learn."**
>
> —Anonymous

Key Terms

Change

Evaluation

Innovation

Measurement

Partnerships

Sustainability

Value

Roles

Communicator

Decision maker

Designer

Educator

Leader

Professional Values

Evidence-based practice

Integrity

Quality

Core Competencies

Anticipation

Communication

Coordination

Design

Project management

Resource management

Introduction

The identification of a meaningful project that guides student learning and impacts clinical practice over time is realized as projects are initiated and completed. This chapter provides the reader with opportunities to review examples of student assignments, information from faculty, and exemplars of student projects. The exemplars provided are **value-**added examples from students who successfully matriculated through executive nurse administration, clinical nurse leader (CNL), and doctor of nursing practice (DNP) programs.

Student projects complement didactic instruction and are common requirements for progression in an executive nurse administration track, a clinical nurse leader track, and a doctor of nursing practice track. While each track has unique requirements, there are specific components that are foundational to all project work. Specific guidelines include:

- Needs assessment
- Gap analysis
- Work flow
- Making the business case

Quality improvement models and evidence-based interventions are included and integrated with these guidelines as students develop, implement, and evaluate project plans. Outlining outcome measures and **evaluation** strategies are also foundational to any project. Specific student assignment components and student project examples for each track that illustrate project components follow.

Executive Nurse Administration Track Project Components

- Project planning, management, and implementation are included in the field study and internship.
- A needs assessment in the form of an organizational analysis is the first step in the project planning process; the results generate the urgency needed to embark on the project.
- In collaboration with a preceptor/mentor, the project idea and business case are developed and aimed at the improvement of care in the meso and/or macrosystem.
- Evidence-based practice (EBP) and quality improvement (QI) are integrated into the project requiring the student to appraise the literature for the strongest research evidence. EBP and QI model inclusion is an expectation.
- Course faculty and the student's preceptor serve as advisors for the student's project. The project serves as a centerpiece of the student's experience, integrating concepts from core and cognates.

- Students select projects that align with strategic plans to facilitate sustainability.
- The student, as project manager, collaborates with preceptors to reinforce leadership, collaboration, and relationship-building skills. Marketing one's work using relationship-based persuasion strategies is an expectation.

Clinical Nurse Leader Track

- The microsystems model serves as a framework for evaluating the five Ps (people, professionals, philosophy [mission], processes, and patterns).
- The immersion experience provides the context for the project plan development and implementation.
- A variety of strategies (evidence-based) that can be implemented within the framework of the project plan are reviewed.
- The cost benefit is cornerstone in making the business case for sustainability of the CNL student's work.

As in the executive nurse administration track, the preceptor is pivotal to success of the student's project, serving as a major stakeholder in championing the project for sustainability. Translating research evidence into a viable quality improvement initiative takes skill and finesse, which further enhances the CNL immersion experience.

Doctor of Nursing Practice Track

- DNP students are expected to develop a systems **change** project.
- A DNP systems change model is provided for students as a guide to developing a project plan.
- The DNP systems change model includes a legend outlining components of the model and appraisal questions.
- Project plan course provides the students the opportunity to have exposure to didactics of project planning.
- Building on the project planning and development course, the student uses Residency I, II, and III to plan, develop, and implement his or her unique systems change project essential to practice.

- Clinical/administrative practice is cornerstone to all aspects of the student's work.
- Given this requirement, the innovative practice project or synthesis project may focus on rural health, academic medical centers, and population-based care.
- The student is guided by a doctor of nursing practice model.
- Content and context are considered with students expected to integrate process mapping and outcomes management into project plan implementation.
- DNP student projects are expected to improve the quality of practice, using sound research evidence to support sustainable improvement changes.

Cost of Caring Project Example, Doctor of Nursing Practice

Overview

In creating an environment and culture of caring, costs should be a consideration. As a graduate nursing student, the need to understand and develop interventions and project proposals that consider the cost of care and how this impacts overall cost of operating a healthcare organization is required. The task is to complete a cost of caring project using the guidelines that follow.

1. Identify a unit, population, or organization of caring. Examples may include a surgical unit, nursing area in a freestanding unit, hospice program, nurse-run clinic, practice group, etc.
2. Define caring. For example, how the care is described, whether there is a standard of care, whether there is a professional practice model, and if so, describe how caring is incorporated in the practice model.
3. Describe how costs are determined based on the variables, procedures, and/or clinical care provided. What formulas or metrics result in costing out caring?
4. Outline your role in facilitating the environment and culture of caring, particularly in light of cost structures and reimbursement issues.

Budget Plan Example for Capstone Project, Doctor of Nursing Practice

Directions

Develop a budget plan for a proposed capstone project using the following questions as a guide.

1. Product/service and the organization
   What are you proposing/what is the statement of purpose?
   What is the product/service?
   How will the product/service further the mission of the organization?
   How will the product/service fit with the organization's strategic plan?
2. Financial plan
   What is/are the operating budget, revenue, and expenses?
   Explain the capital budget as applicable.

DNP Program Development: An Interview With DNP Faculty

Rocky Mountain University of Health Professions

Sandra L. Pennington and Marie Eileen Onieal

1. **Since a project (capstone, systems change, etc.) is required for completing the DNP program, how are students brought along regarding the process? Consider when they begin this work, the number of course hours dedicated to project development, and hours dedicated to implementation, etc.**

Students are encouraged to consider a burning issue in practice needing improvement in light of national needs. Even before the students arrive on campus, faculty challenges the students' typical preconceived notion about the purpose of the capstone project as one of research. Extending this mind-set about the project in the introductory courses and in one-on-one discussions assists students in recognizing that the project is about planned system change that mobilizes healthcare providers to improve healthcare delivery. The 38-credit program draws on course assignments to facilitate project development. Ideally, each student should begin early with a quality improvement idea that can be expanded and redefined in a systematic and self-reflective manner. Faculty encourages a practice issue that coincides with one of the Institute of Medicine's (IOM's) 20 priority areas and the Healthy People 2010 initiatives. Building on the initiative of transforming care at the bedside and the IOM aims for quality (safe, effective, efficient, equitable, patient centered, and timely), faculty emphasize a student's charge of crafting a project that demonstrates safe, effective interventions at the point of care. Coursework is designed to help students structure their capstone focus to enhance the efficiency of the care processes while promoting a team approach.

Two capstone project seminars (3 credits total) are specifically targeted towards the steps of program management. The first seminar provides an overview of project planning, including an introduction to the concepts of project management and developing a mission, vision, goals, and outcomes for the project. The use of an evidence-based practice model to guide the program change is emphasized. The second seminar builds on the first course as the student produces a workable schedule and project controls and evaluation. Final planning of the DNP project occurs, and each student presents the proposed capstone project to faculty and colleagues. Each student finalizes with the program director and clinical mentor his/her plan to structure a change project in advanced practice nursing that is evidence-based and involves applied research at the completion of the didactic work.

Two 4-credit residency requirements are in place. For the specialty residency (80 hours), it is recommended that the student identify evidence to support the change being pursued and work with an identified clinical mentor to begin to develop the project for the capstone. For the policy residency (40 hours), it is recommended that students identify the barriers, stakeholders, and any internal (or external) policies that might impede success at making the change. For the implementation and evaluation phase of the capstone, 10 credit hours are allotted for the project completion and oral defense.

2. Given that there are dedicated project planning and management courses, how are support courses (theory, data, and decision making, etc.) integrated into the final project plan?

Students are required, as part of the project, to identify a theory (change, system, policy, nursing) to guide work. Students determine a theory that drives the intervention and an evidence-based practice system change model that provides structure to the change process. A project timeline and budget development are required for the project proposal. The purpose of the budget is to provide evidence of feasibility and sustainability of the project.

3. Who will be the project advisor? Will there be a committee or a team?

Orientation to the purpose and expectations of the project are critical to the project success. Many members of the team hold the same preconceived notions about the purpose of the capstone as being the development of new knowledge. Faculty has discovered that orientation to the expected outcomes and processes streamline the implementation of the project and mitigate those notions. The student selects a subject matter expert from home settings to serve as a clinical mentor. Clinical mentors are oriented to the expectations of roles and the project. Although faculty expect the student to guide the process as an individual, engagement of the healthcare team with the process change is required.

Currently, the program director serves as the academic advisor. Faculty has begun to ask each other to serve as advisors in areas of content expertise.

4. Is institutional review board approval required?

All students at Rocky Mountain University of Health Professions are required to obtain institutional review board (IRB) approval. Because the purpose of the capstone project differs from research activities, faculty found that the standard IRB application did not fit the project and was often a frustrating activity for the students and the IRB committee, particularly when questions regarding subjects and their recruitment were required to be answered. Additionally, most QI efforts, such as those in a capstone project, do not satisfy the definition of *research* under 45 CFR 46.102(d), and therefore are not subject to the Health and Human Services protection of human subjects regulations. However, in instances where QI activities also accomplish a research purpose, regulations for the protection of subjects in research apply. Additionally, uniform scientific manuscript requirements necessitate that informed consent be indicated in the published article. This requirement has significant implications for reporting the application of best practice.

A task force was established to explore the current form, approval processes, and issues related to using the current research-focused application for the capstone project with the DNP program director, the academic dean, the IRB chairperson, and the IRB manager. A focus with the group was to articulate appropriate terminology in the project description. The efforts of the task force led to the creation of an application for system change form that is submitted for all capstone projects. The form clearly articulates project outcomes, the evidence-based practice model used for the system change, and the justification and evidence to support the project. Projects found to be exempt from human subject protection have notations of such on their approval letter. Unexpectedly, the IRB expressed concerns regarding a few projects related to human subject protection. Since the IRB considers education of the requirements within the role, the IRB manager assists the student, with the collaboration of the program director, to translate the project to the original IRB application. Expanded information about the population participating in the practice change is presented. Those projects undergo an exempt or expedited review. The amended IRB forms and new processes have clarified QI and research outcome differences and have reduced approval delay while ensuring human subject protection.

5. What form should the final product take? Will there be a manuscript or a formal presentation?

The final product takes the same process as a dissertation—students present their work to the program director, other faculty as available, and clinical mentor in a formal setting. Presentations are on campus. The student submits to the program director and the mentor the preliminary draft of the work prior to defending his or her work. Students make changes to the draft that were recommended at the presentation. The final manuscript must be approved by the program director. The student is required to have the manuscript bound and submit the original to the university.

6. What lessons have been learned as the program has evolved?

It is increasingly more important to the students that the university hires DNPs to serve on advisory panels and to teach. When the program began, the pool of nursing professionals with the DNP degree was shallow. That the majority of the faculty did not hold the DNP degree was a concern of many students. As the number of nurses with the DNP degree increases, recruiting faculty from that group is recommended.

Education of faculty, clinical mentors, and the IRB as to the expectations for the capstone project is crucial. As previously mentioned, for many, the concept that the student will not be developing new knowledge was a novel one, and often faculty presented conflicting information regarding the type of work the student would be doing and the look of the final product. Clinical mentors attempted at times to redirect the student to a more research-focused project. Consequently, all constituents were frustrated by the process.

Reference

Robert Wood Johnson Foundation and Institute for Healthcare Improvement. (2001). *Transforming care at the bedside.*

A Voice From a Doctor of Nursing Practice Student

Why a Practice Doctorate for Nurses?

Karen M. Ott

Expectations for clinical practitioners to obtain a doctoral degree have long existed for physicians and dentists and more recently for psychologists, pharmacists, optometrists, audiologists, and physical therapists. There is universal recognition among health professionals that a doctorate is an indicator of the achievement of mastery in one's discipline. Why, then, is there discussion and debate for nursing's recognition for and acceptance of the pursuit of the highest level of scholarly clinical practice, the doctor of nursing practice (DNP)?

The DNP builds upon the foundation begun at the master's level of education: the development of critical thinking and decision-making abilities; skills in both knowledge management and clinical management; and the competencies and knowledge to contribute to a body of evidence that continually advances nursing practice. See **Figure 13-1**.

Incorporating advanced critical thinking and decision-making components, the DNP aims to develop a broader scope of practice potential and an in-depth set of skills that spans the range of healthcare needs from preventive to restorative. This level of advanced clinical preparation will be needed to manage the increasingly complex clinical care of patients with multiple-system diseases that are encountered along the entire continuum of healthcare delivery including hospitals, independent primary care facilities, long-term-care settings, rehabilitation facilities, and the home setting. This level of preparation may ultimately serve as a national platform for autonomous advanced nursing practice (Carlson, 2003).

The DNP prepares practitioners to critically assess and integrate health-related research of all disciplines in an economical and reasonable way, so as to contribute to practice-based evidence, incorporate the findings in the

Figure 13-1   DNP value components.

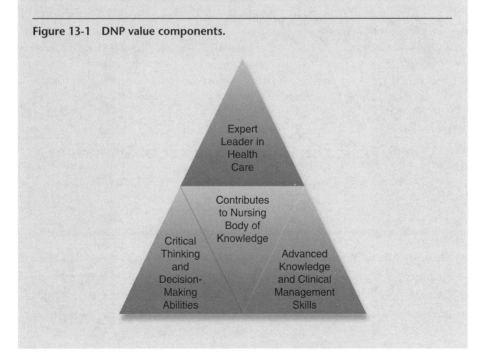

design and development of innovative and improved clinical practice and healthcare delivery models, and evaluate national and global healthcare outcomes (AACN, 2004).

Ultimately, the DNP-prepared practitioner is a healthcare leader whose expertise evaluates and shapes health policy, whose influence and authority drive clinical excellence, and whose principles ensure ethical and exemplary healthcare outcomes. Although it is a demanding and rigorous program of study, the accomplishment of this level of scholarly practice brings personal and professional satisfaction and limitless opportunity for positions of leadership in health care.

Why a practice doctorate for nurses? It's a professionally and personally gratifying course of study; an opportunity to attain professional mastery and an invaluable adjunct to scholarly clinical practice, and it represents an important step for national autonomous nursing practice.

References

American Association of Colleges of Nursing. (2004). *AACN position statement on the practice doctorate in nursing.* Retrieved from: http://www.aacn.nche.edu/DNP/DNPPositionStatement.htm

American Association of Colleges of Nursing. (2009). *Doctor of nursing practice talking points.* Retrieved from http://www.aacn.nche.edu/DNP/talkingpoints.htm

Carlson, L. H. (2003). The clinical doctorate: Asset or albatross? *Journal of Pediatric Health Care 17*(4), 216–218. Retrieved from http://www.medscape.com/viewarticle/458618

Voices From the Field for Master of Science in Nursing Projects

Queens University

Cynthia R. King

The current trend in programs for master's of science in nursing (MSN) is to require students to complete a practicum, research, or evidence-based practice project. The overall goal for these projects is for the student to design, implement, and evaluate a project related to a specialty (e.g., educator, nurse practitioner, healthcare administration, or clinical nurse leader). The majority of nursing programs require that the student complete a scholarly paper and/or professional presentation at the end of the project.

At Queens University in Charlotte, North Carolina, there are three MSN tracks, which include the following: (1) nursing education, (2) healthcare systems administration, and (3) clinical nurse leader. Each student is required to complete a project. Regardless of the track, the projects are called capstone practicum projects. The purpose of the capstone project is to provide the student with the opportunity to apply clinical and theoretical knowledge to a health care-related problem/issue. The selection of a project problem/topic for development must meet the following criteria: (1) the project should concern a problem/topic related to graduate level nursing; (2) there must be a strong emphasis upon related theory and research; (3) the project should offer the student a learning opportunity related to the field of study (education, healthcare system administration, or clinical nurse leader); and (4) the problem or topic should be appropriate to the student's competencies, limits of time, and available resources. The students in the clinical nurse leader program must complete an evidence-based project.

Before starting the project, each student must select a project committee. The committee is composed of a faculty member selected by the student and approved by the chairperson of the master's programs and a preceptor or service/agency representative (from work or a clinical site). The student is encouraged to seek committee members with expertise relevant to the project topic. It is the student's responsibility to obtain the selected members' consent prior to initiating the project. The criteria for preceptors are a nurse with no less than a master's degree in nursing, works at an administrative level higher than the one in which the student is employed, is not in the direct line of authority for the student, and can support student learning congruent with specialty track outcomes.

In collaboration with the faculty and preceptor, students choose a project that can realistically be completed within the time frame of the course. Components of the project are:

1. Clear, measurable objectives
2. A review of relevant and scholarly literature

3. A theoretical framework to guide project implementation
4. Human subjects course and IRB approval, if required
5. An implementation or procedure plan that can be articulated to others
6. Data collection and analyses to evaluate the extent to which project objectives were attained

The capstone project for all three MSN programs results in both a scholarly paper and professional presentation. The student is provided with guidelines for the project that also provide specific headings for the scholarly paper and professional presentation. The student is required to write the paper using the most current American Psychological Association format. The student may present at his/her clinical or work site or at a professional meeting.

Like most MSN programs, Queens University at Charlotte requires students to design, implement, and evaluate a capstone project prior to graduation. Students use the capstone practicum guidelines to understand the criteria for selecting committee members, completing the project, and writing scholarly papers and professional presentation. By the time students complete the project, they have a better understanding of how to apply what was learned in the MSN program to current and future positions.

Practicum Projects of Value: A Successful Strategic Partnership Between Nurse Executives and Master's Level Academia

Joyce A. Hahn

The aging and graying of the nursing workforce extends from the bedside staff nurse to executive management nursing leadership. Availability of educationally prepared nurses to fill the vacancies of the aging and retiring workforce is vital to filling the leadership void for the largest professional discipline in health care. Herrin and Spears (2007) identify, "Without knowledgeable, authoritative nurse leaders at each level of the organization, strategies to improve nursing workforce adequacy, provide safer environments for patients, and manage day-to-day operations of patient care departments cannot be successfully implemented" (p. 231). The purpose of this paper is to describe how one university has formed relationships of collaborative synergy with nurse executives in the metropolitan Washington, D.C., region to provide practicum experiences of value for both the graduate nursing administration students and the healthcare facilities.

An aging workforce study conducted by the Bernard Hodes Group (Hodes Healthcare Division, 2006) in partnership with *Nursing Management* reported 75% of current nurse leaders planned to retire by 2020. Additionally, this survey of 980 nursing leaders from every state in the United States and throughout Canada reported that by 2010 approximately 20% of the nurse leaders will be approaching retirement or already retired. A chief nursing officer (CNO) retention study (Jones, Havens, & Thompson, 2008) reported 62% of respondents anticipated making a job change in less than 5 years with "slightly more than one-quarter for retirement" (p. 89).The data identifies the necessity for senior nursing leadership in the healthcare organizations and master's level academia to form strategic **partnerships** and work collaboratively to prepare the nurse leaders of tomorrow. The George Mason University school of nursing is committed to working with our community healthcare partners to prepare the next generation of nurse leaders. Data from our last three graduating nursing administration classes demonstrates 91% of our students hold nursing administration positions at the director level or higher in the regional area of Washington, D.C.

Academic Partnerships

Academic partnerships with healthcare organizations are not a new paradigm. The rapidly changing healthcare environment, the nursing shortage, and specifically the looming leadership void have resulted in strong partnerships to transform knowledge, skills, and best practices into innovative models and deliverables (Harris & Walters, 2009). The current issues in health care have presented an incentive to forge new relationships of collaborative synergy. Fineout-Overholt, Melnyk, & Schultz (2005) identify collaborative partnerships between academic and healthcare settings as evident in a best-practice culture. The opportunity exists for academia and the nursing executive community to collaboratively create cultures of excellence. This collaborative synergy of intellectually stimulating minds works together to achieve a positive outcome (Kanter, 1989).

The school of nursing at George Mason University welcomes the synergistic partnerships of our community healthcare facilities. The school of nursing vision speaks to educating the next generation of nursing leaders empowered and focused on innovative responses to address the challenges of a rapidly changing and culturally diverse healthcare environment. A recent stakeholder meeting initiated by the director of the school of nursing brought together the nursing executives from our community of healthcare facilities to discuss the needs of the marketplace and how our graduate program could develop, improve, maintain, and assure competent advanced practice nurses.

The master's of science in nursing program is substantial in size, with approximately 300 students. More than one third of this graduate student population is in the nursing administration track. The current curriculum in nursing administration meets the American Association of Colleges of Nursing's (AACN's) *Essentials of Master's Education for Advanced Practice Nursing* (1996), the *Joint Position Statement on Nursing Administration Education* (1997), and the American Nurses Association's (ANA's) *Scope and Standards of Practice for Nurse Administrators* (2004). Each academic year, 25–35 students come together as a cohort for two semesters of nursing administration theory and strategies didactic on campus classroom work and concurrent semesters of practicum experiences (90 hours/semester) with designated nursing administrators. These are the final four courses of the nursing administration track. Prior to these experiences, the students have successfully completed courses in management and organizational theory, financial management, ethics, theoretical foundations in nursing, nursing research methodology, and healthcare delivery systems.

Steps to Practicum Placement

The coordinator for the nursing administration track conducts one-on-one student interviews to discuss each student's anticipated career path and professional goals. Areas of student interest as well as the agency of current employment are identified. Our students are required to complete practicum hours outside of their agency of employment. Each student is requested to submit a set of written goals and expectations for the practicum course sequence. It is at this point that the preceptor match process is initiated.

The coordinator relies upon past preceptors, nursing administration track graduates with two or more years experience in their role, and networking contacts to serve as the potential preceptor pool. Preceptors are required to have an MSN or PhD in nursing and be currently working in an administrative position. Preceptors with strong leadership experience and credentialing are preferred. Practicum sites can include hospital facilities, community-based agencies, professional organizations (e.g., ANA and AONE), health departments, long-term-care facilities, correctional facilities, and entrepreneurial businesses. Students who are novices in the management role are paired with a mid-level administrator, and students with previous relevant nursing management experience are paired with an executive-level administrator.

The coordinator will initiate the contact with the potential preceptor to discuss a possible student placement. The individual student goal statement is e-mailed to the potential preceptor (**Figure 13-2**). Before communication to proceed from the potential preceptor, the student is contacted and a dialogue via telephone or e-mail between the student and preceptor occurs. The preceptor and the coordinator then have a follow-up discussion, and a student practicum

---

Figure 13-2 Sample student goal statement.

By the end of the practicum experience:

- The student will be able to identify one significant project of administrative leadership in alignment with the strategic goals of the organization and the resulting outcome.
- The student will be able to identify at least one challenge of the healthcare organization/unit and the resulting success of implementing evidence-based practice to meet the challenge.
- The student will be able to understand the data, legal, and ethical implications used to drive performance improvement in meeting productivity goals for the organization.

placement is determined or deferred. A practicum course packet inclusive of the course requirements, student contact information, and a student evaluation tool is mailed to the preceptor. A face-to-face meeting between the preceptor, instructor, and student at the preceptor facility occurs prior to the start of the fall semester. The coordinator will continue to be available as a resource to the preceptor, be available for additional on-site meetings as required, and will visit the preceptor at the midterm point of the semester. A final on-site meeting with the coordinator, student, and preceptor occurs at the end of the practicum semester.

Fall as the Big Picture

The fall administrative theory and practicum semesters use the general system theory to examine health-related organizations and nursing administration practice within these organizations. Students are expected to integrate knowledge of environmental influences on the healthcare delivery systems, health policy, and technology. They also analyze internal organizational systems and processes that influence organizational success. Topics include the conceptualization of nursing theories and concepts, organization as systems and systems theory, the art of leadership, change management, strategic management, accountability, legal and regulatory compliance, nursing informatics and organizational structure, and analysis. Students meet weekly on campus as the entire cohort for the theory class and weekly in smaller groups (10–12 students) with an instructor for a seminar-style practicum course. Students are expected to complete 90 hours within this semester with their preceptors. The work product deliverable of the precepted practicum is an organizational analysis paper utilizing the systems theory to identify the links between the theory and the practice within an agency with emphasis on role definition and collaboration among the leadership team at the practicum site. Students will interview members of the leadership team to accomplish this assignment. It is within this first practicum semester that the final practicum project is identified with the preceptor to meet with the practicum project objectives. A practicum project proposal is written to meet the course objectives (**Figure 13-3**) and to meet the identified project need of the nurse administrator and healthcare facility. The project proposal

Figure 13-3   Practicum objectives.

1. Develop a project that relates to the purpose of the practicum assignment, student's interest, and agency's interest and approval.
2. Utilize appropriate administrative and/or nursing theories in development and implementation of the project.
3. Apply appropriate management principles in development and implementation of the project.
4. Utilize research findings as found in the literature.
5. Analyze the impact of nursing service and nursing education conceptual and theoretical formulations within the agency on the project.
6. Evaluate results of the project in terms of purpose and objectives.

(**Figure 13-4**) is reviewed and discussed by both the preceptor and the practicum instructor before the student can proceed with the project. The collaborative synergy of the preceptor, student, and practicum instructor has proven to identify practicum projects of value to the facility and the student's learning experience.

Spring as the How-to Semester

The spring administrative strategies and practicum semester requires the student to integrate theory, research findings, and experience in the analysis of clinical systems, communication frameworks, and interactional processes. Topics include emotional intelligence, managerial and leadership theories in review, evidence-based research and the nursing administrator, conflict resolution, decision making and problem solving, legal and ethical decision making, strategies to effectively manage a multigenerational and diverse staff, human resources, quality management, current topics in health policy and the journey from management to leadership. The spring practicum requires 90 hours/semester of on-site practicum and the weekly campus seminar. Deliverable practicum projects include a seminar presentation of administrative best practice case studies, a managerial work project to demonstrate managerial theory in practice in an actual healthcare setting, and the final practicum project.

Figure 13-4 Sample student practicum proposal.

- **Overview of the Project:** The completed project will address nurse staffing and scheduling, specifically the impact of using 12-hour shifts at Hospital X. The goal is to use data collected during the 3-month trial period to establish measurable evidence-based outcomes to validate this change in staffing patterns.
- **Description of Need:** There is an organizational need to examine the impact of 12-hour shifts on staff productivity, quality of care provided to clients, nursing staff morale, and nursing retention.
- **Project Description:** The data collected will examine the effect of 12-hour shifts on employee satisfaction, productivity, attendance, quality of patient care (medication errors, fall rates, accidents, injuries), impact on other team members, retention rates, impact on recruitment, overtime usage, documentation, and completion. During the postevaluation, data will be examined for its value to the project.
- **Reports Generated:** A written report will be presented to the management team and members of the 12-hour-shift work team. A presentation of results will be given for all nursing staff.
- **Project Timetable:** The project will be completed during the spring semester. The 3-month pilot period for 12-hour shifts started in November, and data collection will begin during the last week of January. An interim report will be presented the first week in March, and a final report will be presented the last week in April.
- **Comments:** Nurse staffing involves different components, including planning, scheduling, and allocation. Scheduling entails assigning nurses for specific time periods by shift (8 hours vs. 12 hours), based on patient care needs. However, by increasing the length of RN shifts administration must be sure that the hours worked in no way pose a threat to patient safety. Hospital X strives to be responsive to staffing needs, retention, and moral issues during a time of national nursing shortages. By introducing a trial period of 3 months for 12-hour shifts and following this up by producing measurable outcomes, any potential for negative patient outcomes can be avoided.

Approved:

Practicum instructor   Date.

Preceptor signature   Date:

Student signature   Date:

Practicum Projects

Student practicum projects can be viewed within the broad categories of quality and safety, business skills, leadership, and strategic planning. All projects must be identified as having value to both the healthcare organization and the student. The student's participation in the project ends at the conclusion of the academic spring semester with a copy of the written project report left with preceptor.

Student practicum project outcomes have been consistently reported by the nursing executives to be of positive value to their organization. A final written student evaluation inclusive of a practicum project rating is submitted by the preceptor. Our nursing administration track over the past 3 years has enjoyed a 100% satisfaction rate with the final practicum project. Open lines of communication between the student, preceptor, and the university faculty over the course of the two semesters beginning with the student goal statement, the mutually agreed-upon practicum proposal, and face-to-face meetings result in positive collaborative and synergistic outcomes.

A brief explanation of the outcomes of the practicum projects is presented in **Table 13-1**. The County Public Health Coalition planning grant and the grant application for system-wide nurse internships were both awarded. A surgical improvement project and the tracking tool for the performance improvement and quality control for compliance are both projects still in place and functioning after the student practicum conclusion. The wound care center opened. The new acute care facility opened, utilizing the transition plan and staff orientation developed by the student. The emergency preparedness spring disaster drill, written by the student with scenarios impacting areas of the hospital from the emergency department to the operating room and all departments in between, was declared a successful first attempt by the organization. The drill was critiqued, updated, and run again just prior to the presidential inauguration to prepare and raise staff awareness. Cultural competency projects in both the local healthcare organization and the professional organization continue. The leadership projects addressing shared governance and working on nursing satisfaction survey issues are moving forward on an organizational basis. The economy and state budget reductions placed the student in a position to use her knowledge and skill sets to assist the healthcare facility in a time of financial crisis. The evaluation of the electronic documentation system aided the organization with its strategic plan initiative to improve patient safety. These were all projects of importance and value.

Table 13-1   Sample Practicum Projects

Practicum Project	Description
Surgical care improvement project	Project based on CMS national standards for reduction of surgical complications by 25%—Medicare reimbursement reduction of 2% if data is not reported.
Performance improvement and quality control for compliance of the Centers for Medicare and Medicaid Services (CMS) detailed notice of discharge regulations	Development of a tracking tool for chart reviews created in response to the new regulation. Compliance monitoring to measure tool effectiveness.
Cultural competency assessment	Hospital-wide cultural competency assessment with analysis, proposal for next steps.
Cultural competency toolbox—national nursing professional organization	Reviewed submissions from state chapters, identified themes, Web page development.
Emergency preparedness: spring disaster drill	Student lead on disaster preparedness committee for drill implementation and outcome analysis.
Mass casualty triage plan	Emergency department response plan in anticipation of pandemic flu or terrorist biologic attack.
Wound care center development	Student developed and presented business plan.
An evaluation of the electronic documentation system	Student measurement and analysis of data.

Table 13-1   Sample Practicum Projects *(continued)*

Practicum Project	Description
Transition to a new acute care facility	Hospital expansion to a new facility in neighboring town. Student provided substantial input to the transition planning process.
County Public Health Coalition planning grant	$20,000 planning grant for mental health services.
Formalized standard for nurse internships	Grant application to a nursing foundation for new system-wide internships.
Lessons learned from litigation	Report prepared utilizing retrospective data research and presentation to facility Medical administrative board and board of directors.
Appreciated inquiry project for shared governance	Preparation of a manual, guidelines, and staff presentations for developing unit and department shared governance.
Budget development and management plan	Resource allocation plan necessary for state hospital facing severe budget cuts.
Action plan to address issues identified in nursing satisfaction survey	Development of an action plan with presentation to nursing management team and hospital CEO.

The nursing administration track coordinator and practicum faculty are available as resources throughout the practicum project process. A final student evaluation of the semester by the preceptor occurs with the coordinator or faculty member at the preceptor's organization. Comments, concerns, and suggestions are all solicited to assist in maintaining a nursing administrative track of high quality to continue meeting the needs of the nursing administrative community. Examples of three practicum project descriptions together with quotes from the student and preceptor are presented in **Table 13-2.**

Table 13-2 Practicum Project Descriptions With Comment

Practicum Project Title: Wound Care Center Business Plan

Evidence-based research conducted with wound care clinics has demonstrated improved patient outcomes, the potential for a decreased hospital length of stay and increased patient satisfaction. The wound care healing center project was undertaken to address the feasibility of bringing such a center to this healthcare organization. A strategic business plan was developed to include market analysis, business operations, and a SWOT analysis.

This project afforded me the opportunity to experience all the components of a new project start-up to include leading an interdepartmental project team and the development of a business plan. C. L., graduate student

The Wound Healing Center business plan was a very well researched plan that examined the competition and internal and external barriers and opportunities and identified the patient population and marketing plan as well as staffing and start-up budget. The work team that the student led brought together many diverse departments within the organization, which enabled the development of a strong sense of mission vision for the project. W. A., associate director of nursing, preceptor

Practicum Project Title: Development of a Nurse Externship Program

The nurse externship program was designed to be used as recruitment and a retention tool to facilitate a smooth transition from the student role to the professional role. Components of the plan involved writing a grant to financially support the program, developing an outline that delineated the program components, planning educational opportunities, and developing a competency checklist and participant evaluations.

Each separate component of the project had unique requirements that collectively have given me valuable insight into program development and grant writing. This experience has instilled in me the confidence to seek out and pursue relevant opportunities for grant writing in my expanding professional career. J. F., graduate student

The value to the organization included the deliverable of an externship project inclusive of evaluation tools for measurement of success. The full value of the project will be determined when we look at the retention rate of this cadre of externs. S. S., director of staff development, preceptor

Table 13.2   Practicum Project Descriptions With Comment *(continued)*

Practicum Project: Emergency Preparedness: Spring Disaster Drill

The goal of the practicum project was to implement a disaster prepared-ness drill to test the emergency operational preparedness at the hospital. The project involved creating realistic threat scenarios with timelines and interjects. The drill was successfully implemented with an immediate critique for strengths and weaknesses by members of the emergency preparedness committee.

Invaluable experience was gained in team leadership and implementation of the disaster drill utilizing the principles of adult learning in relation to theo-ries of chaos and organizational stress. J. I., graduate student

Terrorist attacks, natural disasters, biologic and chemical threats have pushed emergency preparedness to the forefront of hospital agendas. Organized drills testing all levels of preparedness from the day of the incident to recovery phases are necessary. Meeting The Joint Commission emergency management standards and adapting to the hospital incident command structure are required. Our student was tasked to be the project leader, and with members of our emergency preparedness committee, she designed, implemented, and evaluated an exercise that would test our systems and the human response to an external or internal threat. R. F., associate director of nursing, preceptor

Conclusion

The collaborative synergistic model described is a win-win situation for the university and the healthcare facility. The nurse administrator's time commitment is for the 90 hours of precepted time the student spends with the administrator. The student receives additional instruction and mentoring from the university faculty during classroom time. Our program receives networking contacts from interested nursing administrators in our community and is open to new collaborative partnerships. Strategies that might be employed if you are seeking to develop a nurse administrator and university collaboration would include meeting with nurses in your own facility who are attending a college or university to discuss ideas for partnerships and solicit academic contacts; engage in dialogue with nurse administrators in your organization to identify potential preceptors and organizational commitment, then contact the dean of an area college or university to discuss possible collaborative partnerships based on organizational needs and the potential opportunities for preceptors and practicum projects.

The strategic preceptor partnerships described in this descriptive discourse offer graduate students the invaluable opportunity to experience the in-depth, real-world perspective of nursing administration resulting in the enrichment of their academic scholarship. A final practicum work project is designed collaboratively with the preceptor and completed by the end of the second practicum semester. The resulting practicum project is an example of a mutually rewarding experience for the graduate nursing administration student and the preceptor.

References

American Association of Colleges of Nursing. (1996). *The essentials of master's education for advanced practice nursing.* Washington, DC: Author.

American Association of Colleges of Nursing. (1997). *Position statement on nursing administration education.* Washington, DC: Author.

American Nurses Association. (2004). *Scope and standards for nurse administrators.* Washington, DC: Author.

Fineout-Overholt, E., Melnyk, B. M., & Schultz, A. Z. (2005). Transforming health care from the inside out: Advancing evidence-based practice in the 21st century. *Journal of Professional Nursing, 21*(6), 335–344.

Harris, J. L., & Walters, S. E. (2009). Building a portfolio for academic and clinical partnership. In L. Roussel, with R. C. Swanburg (Eds.), *Management and leadership in nursing administration* (5th ed., pp. 608–617). Sudbury, MA: Jones and Bartlett.

Herrin, D., & Spears, P. (2007). Using nurse leader development to improve nurse retention and patient outcomes. *Nursing Administration Quarterly, 31*(3), 231–243.

Hodes Healthcare Division. (2006). *The 2006 aging workforce study.* Atlanta, GA: The Bernard Hodes Group.

Jones, C. B., Havens, D. S., & Thompson, P. A. (2008). Chief nursing officer retention and turnover: A crisis brewing? Results of a national survey. *Journal of Healthcare Management, 53*(2), 89–106.

Kanter, R. M. (1989). *When giants learn to dance* (pp. 36, 114, 153–155). New York: Simon & Shuster. Sample student practicum proposal.

Executive Nurse Administration Exemplars

Implementation of a Perioperative Efficiency Program

Amy Beard

Problem Statement

Efficiency and productivity are essential to successful businesses, including healthcare organizations; however, there is no consensus on how to define it nor the best approach to sustain efficiency in perioperative areas. Wasted time is wasted money. Inefficient operating rooms equate to lost revenue-generating opportunities for all involved (Surgery Management Improvement Group, 2009). This provided the impetus to implement a perioperative efficiency program. The program goals were to achieve 80% compliance with established utilization targets, limit case cancellations to a maximum, and achieve a turnaround time of 20 minutes from case to case.

Knowledge Gap

Efficiency in perioperative areas is widely examined by others, yet no consensus for how to define efficiency has been reached. While a wide range of solutions for improving efficiency in the perioperative area is cited in the literature, more longitudinal studies are needed to validate the best solutions for implementation (Arakelian, Gunningberg, & Larsson, 2008; Zheng, Martinec, Cassera, & Swanstrom, 2008).

Team Development and Inclusion

Riley and Manias (2005) recommended that perioperative efficiency is best accomplished by improving coordination between and among team members. Heslin and colleagues (2008) supported this notion that implementation of data-driven changes in short, immediate, and long-term strategies are realized when multidisciplinary team members are engaged. These provided guidelines for team inclusion to effect change and attain targets.

Project Processes

The plan, do, study, act (PDSA) model for improvement provided the foundation for a series of actions directed at achieving the project goals. When applying the PDSA model to improve efficiency, two main components are considered. First are the questions that drive the process improvement team; and second, the plan-do-study-acts that allow improvement in processes to be evaluated in a real environment. The team determines opportunities for improvement that are evidence based and then tests the primary tenets of an idea on a small scale. Central to this project were the following objectives:

1. Implement a perioperative efficiency program to improve patient outcomes.
2. Seek as many opportunities as possible for improving efficiency.
3. Using lean methodologies, improve efficiencies as evidenced by 80% compliance with perioperative utilization methods, reduced case cancellations, and achievement of a turnaround time from case to case of 20 minutes.

Direct communication and education with surgeons and operating room staff continuously occurred throughout the improvement process.

Evaluation Methods

A series of activities were developed and implemented in order to evaluate the improvements. For increased utilization compliance, the actions included the following:

1. Relocation of the utilization area
2. Targeted communication with providers with low utilization rates
3. Education of providers on utilization as related to same-day procedures
4. Documentation of nonutilization on the surgical board by provider
5. Review of the surgery schedule in advance to arrange scheduling for enhanced flow

Evaluation improvement activities to meet the objective of reducing case cancellations occurred by the following:

1. Tracking reasons by provider, group, and patient
2. Developing action plans based on findings using the PDSA model
3. Evaluating utilization as a predictor of surgery cancellations
4. Evaluating use of proxies as a predictor of surgery cancellations
5. Establishing a definition for case cancellation to assure data integrity
6. Focusing on four primary case cancellations reasons

To ensure evaluation of the turnaround objective was met, the following strategies were included.

1. Communication with the multidisciplinary team
2. Staff and provider education on turnaround definition and goal
3. Improvement of inventory supply management
4. Improvement of communication among all surgical areas

Outcomes

Based on this improvement intervention, operating room efficiency increased and cost savings were realized. More specifically, the following outcomes occurred.

Cost Savings From Improved Efficiency

- Increased total operating minutes
- Increased gross margin per case

Additional Opportunities Realized by the Project

- Increased utilization rates for the perioperative area
- Missed opportunity found by reducing turnaround time to 20 minutes, thus increasing volume
- Evidence to support more cases could occur based on the current 24 cases per day (increasing to 32) and data to support the revenue that could be generated by the increase

This project is one example of the value of using a model to guide change and the involvement of multiple team members in accomplishing goals. Data-driven change should be the ultimate goal of any initiative.

References

Arakelian, E., Gunningberg, L., & Larsson, J. (2008). Job satisfaction or production? How staff and leadership understand operating room efficiency: A qualitative study. *Acta Anaesthesioligical Scandinavica, 52*(100), 1423–1428.

Heslin, M. J., Doster, B. E., Daily, S. L., Waldrum, M. R., Boudreasu, A. M., & Smith, A. B. (2008). Durable improvements in efficiency, safety, and satisfaction in the operating room. *American College of Surgeons, 20*, 1083–1089.

Institute for Healthcare Improvement. (2009). *Setting aims.* Retrieved from http://www.ihi.org/IHI/Topics/Improvement/ImprovementMethods/How/ToImprove/setting+aims.htm

Riley, R., & Manias, E. (2005). Governing times in operating rooms. *Journal of Clinical Nursing, 15*, 546–553.

Scheriff, K., Gunderson, D., & Intelisano, A. (2008). Implementation of an OR efficiency program. *AORN, 88*(5), 775–789.

Surgery Management Improvement Group. (2009). *Rapid operating room turnover.* Retrieved from http://www.surgerymanagement.com/presentations/rapid-operating-room-turnover1.php

Zheng, B., Martinec, D. V., Cassera, M. A., & Swanstrom, L. L. (2008). *Surgical Endoscopy, 22*, 2171–2177.

Changing the Model of Care

Sharon Cusanza

Problem Statement

Practice is best guided by a consistent model, and within a healthcare system with multiple sites, it is essential. For facilities that are designated as a Magnet organization, a professional model of care, based upon a theory, must be adopted and operationalized (ANCC, 2008). Only one of the six organizations with a multisite healthcare system has had a model of care for the past 17 years. In that organization, the current professional model of care is not congruent with a theoretical model nor is it applicable to all patient care areas throughout the organization.

Knowledge Gap

With the change in the Magnet standards and the growth of the multisite system, nursing management decided that it would be a good time to initiate this major change. As a result of participation in a journal club with the system nursing executive council, it was decided to utilize relationship-based care in the new model, as posed by Koloroutis (2004).

Team Development and Inclusion/Project Processes

Changing the model of care is usually a long-term project. However, this project was divided into three phases for accomplishment over a 12- to 18-month time frame. Phase one was a project to meet course requirements. Phases two and three became part of an evolving role in a paid position.

Phase one consisted of several initiatives. Focus groups were conducted on each campus for stakeholder acceptance (Kotter, 1995). Nursing councils were used for focus groups whenever possible. Following an explanation of the intended goal, displaying the tenets of the model whenever possible, general feedback along with targeted questions about how to create urgency and identify and overcome potential barriers were elicited. Feedback was incorporated into the plan. Most of the feedback applied to the way to present the model to staff. These ideas were incorporated into the model and used to inform the staff.

The next initiative was to implement the kickoff celebration during Nurses' Week. A survey of staff revealed that most nurses wanted to receive education hours during the weeklong celebration. A continuing nursing education program that included two guest speakers focusing on relationship-based care was developed and offered. With the assistance of media production staff, an inspirational video to introduce the tenets of the new model was produced.

The caring model (Dingman, Williams, Fosbinder, & Warnick, 1995) is based on linkage of five actions to improve patient satisfaction. One of the major parts of the caring model is sitting at the bedside at eye level with the patient to discuss the plan of care for the day. The executive and management teams granted permission and set the expectation of the staff to take this action using tools provided to assist them. Posters and pocket cards were provided as cues.

Lastly, a name-the-model contest occurred so the staff could create a name and develop a pictorial representation of the model, thus engaging others—a shared governance strategic action. The contest was advertised among staff and 10 entries were received. The executive team review resulted in selection of five entries for voting by staff.

Evaluation Methods and Outcomes

Following the implementation of the model, a decision was reached to compare patient satisfaction scores from the medical/surgical units as an equitable comparison. Data from the Press Ganey patient satisfaction survey, a valid and reliable tool, was reviewed preimplementation (in April) and postimplementation (in June) of the model. Overall satisfaction increased from 86.6% to 87.6%. In addition, nursing staff were surveyed before and after model implementation about relationship-based care. Data were collected three different times within a 3-month period. Due to the short survey period, response rates for the last query were lower. Using a chi-square test resulted in no significant differences on any of the questions asked with the exception of one, "True or false: when I was providing care to my patients, they were at the center of my attention." The significance was calculated at p = 0.47.

References

American Nurses Credentialing Center. (2008). *The Magnet recognition program application manual*. Silver Spring, MD: Notebooks.

Dingman, S., Williams, M., Fosbinder, D., & Warnick, M. (1995). Implementing a caring model to improve patient satisfaction. *Journal of Nursing Administration, 38*(4), 172–177.

Koloroutis, M. (Ed.). (2004). *Relationship-based care: A model for transforming practice*. Minneapolis, MN: Creative Health Care Management.

Kotter, J. (1995). Leading change: Why transformation efforts fail. *Harvard Business Review, 73*(2), 59–67.

Analysis of the Nurse Hiring Process

Traci Solt

Problem Statement

Delays in hiring nurses result in inadequate staffing and can have an adverse impact of the quality of care, employee morale, and the bottom line (Government Accountability Data [GAO], 2008). The project was aimed at identifying factors that contributed to delays in hiring registered nurses (RNs) at a complex, multisite federal medical center.

Knowledge Gap

Limited data were available to support the proposition that a standardized process of hiring employees using a tracking system will streamline the process and delay gaps in employing staff. Utilizing the evidence hierarchy posed by Polit and Beck (2008) and the GOA data, the knowledge gap was reduced, thus assisting in developing the project process and goal.

Although the data does not include a high level of evidence hierarchy, a gap in the process that required additional investigation was identified. Information related to timelines in the nurse hiring process was obtained via survey data and interviews. Best practices from other facilities (federal and local community) were reviewed, as was an activity directed at reducing the knowledge gap.

Team Development and Inclusion

Collaboration, communication, and coordination among leadership and human resources management are required in order to reduce hiring delays. This was supported from the findings of this project.

Project Processes and Evaluation Methods

Assessment

A tracking tool was created utilizing the process map. In an effort to identify any common themes related to the hiring process, interviews and surveys followed with stakeholders.

Because of the lack of strong evidence related to time frames for hiring new nurses, this author compared the current process to that of a similar federal healthcare facility. The data revealed reduction of delays in the hiring process as a result of specific actions and interventions. Although the level of evidence from the literature is sparse, this author postulated the data were strong evidence that the recommendation for the project would succeed in reducing delays in the hiring process.

Measurement

Process maps of the nurse hiring process were created to identify each step. The first process map illustrated 18 steps in the hiring process from approval to fill the position to the first day of employment. This process was too large in scope to examine and investigate, and the project was narrowed to consider the process from tentative selection to firm offer, which was a new performance metric that had been identified by the facility. A swim lane process map was created to drill down to each individual step. The map identified three rework loops, two of which were be considered for intervention.

Financial Impact

It is estimated that continued delays will cost one facility $38,000 per month and more at others dependent on locality pay scales. This is attributed to overtime pay, decreased morale, and the loss of physician staff due to lack of nursing support for care delivery to patients.

Implementation

The data collected and process maps were used to determine root causes and opportunities for improvement. Critical drivers of the defects were:

- Lack of tracking mechanisms
- No standardization
- Conflicting issues related to validation of credentials
- Complicated instructions to complete the hiring process

Outcomes

Although there is strong evidence to support implementation of the processes that can reduce the time frame for hiring staff and reduce associated costs, successful integration will require extensive collaboration between nursing and human resources. The bureaucratic nature of the organization produced obstacles in the implementation phase. Barriers related to the organizational structure of the facility included the following silos:

- Administrative and support services
- Patient care services
- Medicine services

The two key players in this process included nursing and human resources; each service is located in different silos. Leadership for each silo is managed by an executive leadership team. This process is inefficient and poses enormous obstacles to success.

While participation in this performance improvement process was painstaking and eye opening, it provided information related to interorganizational communication. Process mapping is a useful tool as evidenced in this project.

References

Government Accountability Office. (2008). *VA health care: Improved staffing methods and greater availability of alternate and flexible work schedules could enhance the recruitment and retention of inpatient nurses (GAO-09-17)*. Washington, DC: U.S. Government. Retrieved from www.gao.gov/highlights/d0917high.pdf

Pilot, D., & Beck, C. (2008). *Nursing research: Generating and assessing evidence for nursing practice* (8th ed.). Philadelphia: Lippincott Williams & Wilkins.

Hughes Spalding Clinic Improvement

Julie Tragott

Problem Statement and Team Inclusiveness

In 2006, Children's Healthcare of Atlanta (Children's), managing the Hughes Spalding Campus, planned to rebuild the entire hospital to meet the needs of the underserved pediatric populations in Georgia. Shortly after Children's decided to do this, the nation rapidly experienced an economic decline that led Children's leaders to reexamine what services were productive to maintain viability. It was decided that if the Hughes Spalding Pediatric Clinic continued to decrease in volume, there could be a reduction in the number of clinic beds Children's could offer. For many Atlanta families, this clinic was the only healthcare resource. The project was not just about making a difference or improving care to this population. Many children would likely go without care if drastic initiatives were not immediately begun.

Knowledge Gap

Evidence of hierarchy was used to rank evidence sources according to the strength of the evidence's methodology, clinical relevance, and reliability (Pilot & Beck, 2008). This information provided opportunities to not only review relevant literature for use, but also to note the absence of literature and strategies that could be incorporated into the processes confronting redesign/ changes needed in services for viability.

Project Processes and Evaluation Methods

The Hughes Spalding Pediatric Primary Clinic Improvement Initiative's overall purpose was to improve patient accessibility, throughput, and volumes, as well as clinic performances and satisfaction. This project was initiated using the project management body of knowledge phases as posed by Lewis (2007) and that include the following.

- Initiate
- Plan
- Execute
- Monitor and control
- Evaluate/control

Phase I: Initiate

The pediatric primary care clinic project was selected based on an operational desire to improve patient throughput, volumes, and satisfaction. The key stakeholders were identified, met, and agreed to be active members in the initiation phase. Weekly meetings were arranged to determine clinic needs, project objectives, and the desired long-term goals. The team obtained initial project approval from the vice president of operations, who agreed to be the leadership champion.

Phase II: Plan

During the planning phase, baseline **measurements** were established by performing a patient/family survey, determining current no-show rates, and conducting patient throughput time studies. The team completed a lean process development course to increase knowledge on how to reduce wasted resources and streamline throughput flow. The team identified and documented goals, scope, tasks, and schedules and estimated costs, risks, quality, and staffing needs. The team agreed upon organizational planned commitments to initiate and establish a baseline of the plan from which the project was managed.

Phase III: Execute

Scheduling The task force reviewed all exiting schedules to transition into an open-access hybrid with the goal to assist with improving no-show rates for both scheduled and walk-in patients. The team developed a new schedule that allowed patients to merge into the mid-level provider's appointment schedule, thereby eliminating a separate clinic. A proposed schedule was presented to the team prior to going live.

Registration The task force identified opportunities to more quickly register patients to get them to an exam room. The intent was to benefit flow when an influx of patients arrived. Intake forms were redesigned and placed strategically in clinic areas. Each exam room was standardized with the same equipment, and processes to improve processing of claims also occurred.

Triage The task force developed nursing process change to assist clinic techs triage. A new nursing model was introduced with defined roles for team, lead roles, and lab logs.

Patient Flow The team reviewed and created new chart forms. All exam rooms were set up to mirror supplies and equipment. This enhanced flow and reduced patient wait times.

Provider Exams The team developed an access program time study database to monitor, trend, and control patient travel times through the clinic. Benchmark data were used to set goals for providers to improve patient flow and assessment practice. The findings were presented at provider team meetings.

Operational Process Improvement The team developed a new component, back office, and staffed it with a nurse to assist internal and external communication that included the following: a prescription refill phone line, consultation reports and faxes, immunization documentation requests, and demographic information completion.

Phase IV: Monitor and Control

Predata were collected prior to implementing the new processes and included the following:

- No-show rate metrics 37.9%
- Customer services survey 89.9%
- Nursing engagement survey
- Throughput time metrics 103 minutes
- Budget volume and variance metrics 20%, negative net volume

Phase V: Evaluate Goals Timeline

April, September, and December were the identified months for evaluation of goal attainment.

Outcomes

- No-show rates decreased by 7.9%
- Customer service scores increased by 4.1%
- Nursing engagement survey increased by 16%

- Patient throughput time decreased by 18 minutes
- Budget volumes increased by 20%

Health care is characterized by increasing patient demand, constrained staffing and physical resources, and rising cost of capital. Optimizing patient throughput has become an essential operations management strategy for nurse executives. The goal is to provide efficient use of resources and have a high return on revenues. Optimized patient throughput promotes savings in capital and revenue growth opportunities. Most importantly, optimized inpatient throughput enhances patient access, reduces clinic cost, and improves the quality of care and services provided.

References

Lewis, J. P. (2007). *Fundamentals of project management*. New York: American Management Association.

Polit, D., & Beck, C. (2008). *Nursing research: Generating and assessing evidence for nursing practice* (8th ed.). Philadelphia: Lippincott Williams & Wilkins.

CNL Project Exemplars

Fall Reduction Project Plan

Drew Glazner

Problem Statement and Team Inclusion

The deleterious effects and costs associated with falls demand action. The costs for care related to a patient fall within the hospital setting will no longer be covered by insurance; these costs will fall on the care facility in which the incident occurred. If the fall results in an increase in stay, it could cost the hospital $1,000/day for room and daily supplies alone. Knowledgeable of such, the fall committee at a large urban healthcare trauma facility used evidence to introduce interventions to reduce falls, such as the introduction of new bed alarms.

The project sought to answer the following clinical question. How can inpatient falls be reduced in the adult acute care setting on an identified unit as compared to the national standard fall rate of 3.6 per 1000 patients, with the desired outcome of zero falls with injury?

Knowledge Gap

Observations provide evidence that a significant gap exists in patient rounds during shift turnover. It can take up to 4 hours to receive report from the departing shift, begin patient assessments, and deliver morning medications. Patient falls can and do occur during this time period. Introducing bedside reporting may decrease the time for care delivery and establish a quicker response to patients, thus preventing falls. Interviews with patients were conducted randomly between September and November 2008, and results showed a severe gap in patient education on fall prevention. Of 76 patients interviewed, 65% claimed to have had no previous education on fall risks, and 25% had not been identified as a fall risk but qualify under the fall risk evaluation tool. The IOM defines quality as the level in which healthcare agencies increase the chances of desired outcomes and remain current and consistent within their professional practice (IOM, 2008). This suggests that healthcare organizations should constantly be researching and evaluating new evidence-based practices and ideas for implementation in the effort to improve their quality of care. The IOM initiated the Redesigning Health Insurance Performance Measures, Payment, and Performance Improvement Project in September of 2004. This pay-for-performance project no longer requires insurance agencies to pay for nosocomial infections, pressure ulcers acquired while receiving treatment in an acute care setting, ventilated associated pneumonia, and injuries resulting from falls. These costs are now the responsibility of the facility in which they occurred (IOM).

A literature review was conducted and found several plans in the reduction of patient falls. Increasing staff exposure time to patients by conducting hourly rounds and implementing the three P rule (position, potty, and pain), the Medical Center of Plano, Texas, saw a decrease in patient falls and call light use while increasing its patient satisfaction scores (Leighty, 2007). Hourly rounds and patient/staff education on fall risks were executed at the Mayo Clinic Hospital in Phoenix, Arizona, resulting in a decrease in falls between September 2007 and October 2007 (Charles, Johns, & Yoder, 2008). Reeducation of staff on fall risk identification and hourly rounds were the foci used at the Central Arkansas Veterans Healthcare System, which resulted in a fall rate of zero for the month of July 2008 (Watson, 2008). The final stage of the Iowa evidence-based practice model will be the employment of the new fall reduction protocol and its evaluation on outcomes in the change in practice patterns.

Project Processes and Evaluation Methods

Preevaluation Method and Tools

Bedside reporting was changed to begin at shift change outside of the patient's room and conducted using the demographics, assessments, treatments, alerts, and status sheet. Hourly rounds were slated to consist of assessing the patient's needs for pain, position, possessions, potty, and pumps. Each patient was to receive a yellow call, don't fall education sheet when admitted to the unit to begin his or her teaching process on fall risks. An evaluation tool has been generated to dissect the cause and impact of any falls that occur. Success was to be measured through the use of the evaluation tool and a noted decrease in the amount of falls occurring on the floor.

Implementation

Project education and implementation began early January 2009. Guidelines for bedside reporting were reviewed with the staff during a group meeting and then on a one-to-one basis as needed. Hourly rounds were already in progress, but only for patients labeled as fall risks. Staff were informed that the new protocol for hourly rounds would include all patients and be performed by both RNs and ancillary staff. Patient education cards were laminated and hung in plain sight in each patient room. Staff was informed of the need to take the cards each shift and review them with their patients to reinforce the seriousness of fall reduction and help the patients remember causes of falls. Benefits from bedside reporting include enhanced communication between oncoming and departing shifts, increased RN accountability for current patient and room conditions, increased exposure time to patients, early start on patient assessment and prioritization, decreased costs for overtime accrued at shift change, and increased patient satisfaction and safety. Benefits of hourly rounds include a consistent continuum of care, meeting patient needs in a timely manner, decreased call light usage, increased exposure time, and increased patient satisfaction and safety. Benefits from the call, don't fall placards include a continued reminder of fall prevention for patients; increasing patient education on safety, medication, and equipment; enhanced communication with patients; and increased patient satisfaction and safety.

Outcomes

Who fell? Transforming care at the bedside measure collection sheet for the unit resulted in a decrease in falls from October 2008 to December 2008 (20 falls prior to project implementation) to mid-January 2009 through March 2009, when there were 12 falls. There were 5 falls with injury prior to project implementation while only 1 was recorded after the project start-up (Pomrenke, 2009). The 12 falls break down as follows according to the fall evaluation tool: seven females between the ages of 21 and 82, five males between the ages of 40 and 62; 3 falls occurred at the end of January, 3 falls during the month of February, and 6 during March. Reasons for the falls included one pain issue, one possession (reaching for cell phone), five potty issues, and five position issues. Five of the falls occurred to alert patients, four of whom were not previously labeled as a fall risk, while seven were confused and/or disoriented; all of these seven were previously labeled as a risk. All of the patients who fell had received prior education on fall prevention and their hourly round sheets were completed. The one injury that occurred was an abrasion to the left knee of a 62-year-old male; cost to the hospital was a one-time 4 × 4 and Kerlix dressing and an X-ray of the knee costing $70. In another fall, the final cost to the hospital was a $500 computed tomography of the head from a 41-year-old female who fell due to dizziness from pain medication and complained of a headache; no injury was found.

Staff and patients have reported positive results from hourly rounds and bedside reporting. Nurses have stated, "Noise levels on the unit are down," and "Patients don't ring (call lights) as much now that we are more visible." Patients have communicated a more relaxed feeling during interviews and like the extra attention. Nursing overtime steadily trended down from 132 hours/month to 115 hours/month with a goal of further reduction (Pomrenke, 2009).

Patient safety is a core measure at this facility. Decreasing the inpatient fall rate will be a continued goal for the fifth floor. The patient fall committee and patient safety subcommittee have initiated steps to adhere to best practice interests on fall reduction. The use of nonskid slippers, lowboy beds, and review of the fall risk assessment tool have been initiated during this fall reduction initiative. Continued reevaluation of the microsystem and research of evidence-based practice will be the goal of the clinical nurse leader.

References

Charles, J., Johns, M., & Yoder, A. (2008, November). Patient fall prevention program. Paper presented at the meeting of Transforming Care at the Bedside, San Francisco, CA.

Institute of Medicine. (2008). *Crossing the quality chasm: The IOM health care quality initiative*. Retrieved from http://www.iom.edu/CMS/8089.aspx

Leighty, J. (2007). *Time well spent*. Retrieved from http://include.nurse.com/apps/pbcs.dll/article?AID=200761222015

Peterson, M. (2008). *Inpatient unit profile*. University of South Alabama Medical Center.

Pomrenke, B. (2009). *TCAB measure collection sheet*. Fifth floor unit data, October 2008 through March 2009.

Rapid Modeling. (2008). *Transforming care at the bedside measure collection sheet*. Unit 5, University of South Alabama Medical Center.

Watson, M. (2008, November). *Central Arkansas Veterans Healthcare System: Successful prevention of fall injuries*. Paper presented at the meeting of Transforming Care at the Bedside, San Francisco, CA.

Failure to Rescue

Susan Thomas

Problem Statement

Rapid response teams (RRT) is a system approach that promotes early and appropriate intervention in the care of critically ill patients. According to Aleccia (2009), failure to rescue claimed 188,000 lives between 2004 and 2006. This accounts for 128 deaths for every 1,000 patients who are at risk for complications. These deaths are caused by oversights of healthcare professionals who come in contact with patients during their hospitalization. These oversights include overmedication, poor communication, lack of knowledge, poor assessment skills, and not trusting instincts. RRT, patient advocacy, and communication are three interventions that can be initiated to dramatically decrease the deaths from failure to rescue. The goal of this project was to decrease code blues outside the intensive care unit by 50%, reach patients before critical events occurred, and increase patient and family awareness to have a voice in plans of care.

Knowledge Gap

So what does failure to rescue mean to the healthcare team and can knowledge gaps be filled to eliminate near misses and untoward events? While a variety of data and mandates are drivers for facilities to initiate activities to reduce near misses and catastrophic events, knowledge gaps and variability in approaches exist.

Team Development and Inclusion

When the RRT is called, the nurses are expected to have vital information available. Communication among staff is requisite for positive outcomes. However, development of the RRT requires input from a variety of staff, and input should be incorporated when developing the processes and evaluating outcomes.

Project Processes and Evaluation Methods

An evaluation of rapid responses and codes by nursing floors was initiated. Interviews with RRT members, nursing floor staff, and nurse managers began in an effort to evaluate current issues and individual opinions on what changes could improve the RRT and outcomes. A review of medical records and code forms also occurred to ascertain additional information that could be used to assist in improving outcomes, reducing codes, and including patients and families in plans of care. A new code form was developed and became a part of daily nurse manager duties to identify potential deficits that could reduce or eliminate codes.

Outcomes

By using a systems approach that promotes early and appropriate intervention in the care of critically ill patients, it was anticipated that codes would be reduced by 50%, thereby reducing mortality rates and decreasing length of stays in the intensive care units. Analysis of benefits and barriers to decreasing knowledge gaps and improvement of RRT interventions continued, and lessons learned could guide education of staff, patients, and families. The data from continuous analysis and interventions were expected to drive changes in practice. Preliminary data that supported RRTs as a continuous quality initiative are shown in **Figure 13-5**.

Figure 13-5   RRT/Codes by year.

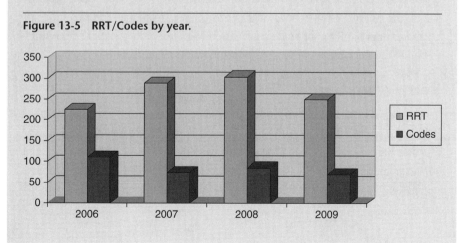

Reference

Aleccia, J. (2009). *Before Code Blue: Who's minding the patient?* Retrieved from http://www.msnbc.msn.com/id/24002334

Doctor of Nursing Practice Exemplars

Pressure Prevention Project

Henri Brown

Problem Statement

Pressure ulcers are a major healthcare problem in hospitalized patients in the United States. Lyder (2003) estimated that annually, 2.5 million patients are treated for pressure ulcers, and approximately 60,000 of them die as a result of complications associated with those pressure ulcers. Even though clinical practice guidelines for prevention and treatment of pressure ulcers exist, many agencies have not incorporated those guidelines into their standard of care.

Lyder (2003) estimated the cost of treating a single grade 3 or 4 pressure ulcer at $70,000; the cost per year for the United States is $1.3 billion. These costs have resulted in a significant financial burden on healthcare systems across the nation. The purpose of this project was to reduce the incidence of pressure ulcers among an acute care patient mix, including critical care units, to below the national mean at an academic health center.

Knowledge Gap

This academic health center was experiencing a pressure ulcer rate of 7.8%, which was higher than the national mean of 7%. A needs assessment indicated that the high incidence was related to prolonged patient stays on hard, flat surfaces, inconsistent skin assessments for patients at risk to develop pressure ulcers, and an inconsistent documentation and follow-up of identified patients at risk.

Team Development and Inclusion

Early in the process, the DNP student identified a mentor who, along with faculty advisors, guided the makeup and development of the team as well as the project as a whole. In this case, the mentor was the wound care clinical nurse specialist for the facility. Other members of the team included a unit champion on each unit, a registered dietician, a physical therapist, and course faculty. This team provided system knowledge as well as professional knowledge to the process. Team members assessed the feasibility and efficacy of the tools developed by the DNP student and provided significant support in the refinement and revision of the project.

Project Processes

The DNP student, an experienced acute care nurse, identified a perceived need for intervention related to pressure ulcers. After conferring with hospital administration, the student performed a comprehensive needs assessment and developed a staged intervention. IRB approval was accomplished as a part of the planning for the needs assessment.

The needs assessment included developing, administering, and evaluating a pretest for nurses and nursing assistants on the causes and methods of preventing pressure ulcers; a detailed observation of the current practices of nurses and nursing assistants in areas where large numbers of patients were experiencing pressure ulcers; and a chart review on all patients who were diagnosed with a pressure ulcer on those units. The pretest results indicated that nursing staff and nursing assistants were not fully aware of the clinical practice guidelines related to pressure ulcers, had not integrated them into their daily routines, and did not understand how their actions or inactions had a direct effect on incidence of pressure ulcers.

The direct observation provided a hospital-wide snapshot of the state of the art with regard to prevention of pressure ulcers. The presence or absence of surface supports on patient beds; the number and type of devices used in positioning patients, such as multiple sheets, rolls, etc., placed on patient beds; the frequency of skin assessments; the presence of a protective barrier for patients who were incontinent of bladder or bowel; and multiple other items comprised this aspect of the needs assessment. The intensive care areas of this particular facility had the largest incidence of pressure ulcer development. Staff and wound care specialists theorized with the DNP student that some of the incidents may reflect poor nutrition for comatose or trauma patients. Another aspect of care was that in trauma cases, frequently there was no cervical spine clearance physician order, causing nurses to be reticent to reposition patients for fear of causing further physical damage.

Chart reviews yielded several examples that validated the findings on the pretest and during direct observation. Documentation of the required Braden scores each shift was not evident; nutritional consultations were not documented, either as needed or completed; and the use of airflow mattresses and pads was not documented. Frequently there was no indication that wound care specialists were notified of the risk factors presented by the patient, even though the risk factors themselves were very evident in the chart and physical therapy consultations were not sought to provide passive or active range of motion for bed-bound patients. The results of the chart audit were alarming, but not unexpected given the direct observation experience.

These results indicated fragmentation in prevention of pressure ulcers, poor documentation of skin assessment and any subsequent action, and lack of integration of evidence-based protocols. Based on this comprehensive, multifocal needs assessment and workflow analysis, the DNP student devised an evidence-based pressure ulcer prevention protocol and the implementation of a coordinated staff education plan. This plan consisted of several phases.

Phase I

The goals of the first phase were to educate nursing and nursing assistant staff on the clinical practice guidelines associated with preventing pressure ulcers; develop chart audit tools for the nurses to use to follow up on protocol adherence; and identify unit-based champions who would reinforce the prevention measures with staff, patients, and families.

Phase II

The goals of the second phase were to develop a nurse-driven, functional screening for pressure ulcers that was comprehensive and feasible; test the chart audit tool for usefulness and embed it as a part of orientation for all new staff; develop a protocol for weekly patient skin assessments; develop a reward system to enhance communication between nursing staff and nursing assistants so that assistants felt included and responsible for daily skin assessments; and integrate allied health professionals into an overall plan to reduce the incidence of pressure ulcers in the entire facility.

Phase III

In phase III, the DNP student assessed plan for **sustainability**, feasibility, and results.

Evaluation Methods

The chart audit tool shown at the end of the case study used to assess for compliance was developed as a part of this project and is currently being used in the facility. A posttest indicated a significant improvement in nurse and nursing assistant knowledge about preventing pressure ulcers and their role in the process. Documentation of the use of the Braden scale in skin assessment is 100% and has remained at that level for a sustained period. The cost savings was demonstrated to hospital administration ($70,000 for treatment of a pressure ulcer or $10 per day for an air flow mattress), and new protocols ensure that an air flow or waffle mattress is used on all patients whose Braden scale score is less than 16 (indicating a patient at risk).

Outcomes

Within the first 3 months, the incidence of pressure ulcers dropped from 7.8% to less than 3%. Sustained reduction of the incidence occurred over the subsequent 3 months. At the end of 6 months, the incidence of pressure ulcers had fallen to 1% of high risk patients, and that figure has been sustained over the past 2 years.

Distinct aspects of the accomplishment of the reduction in incidence of pressure ulcers bear detailed description. For instance, as a direct result of this program, registered dieticians now review charts to ascertain if a prealbumin level has been reported on all patients at risk of developing a pressure ulcer. If a level exists, the dietician uses the prealbumin to determine the protein content of the patient's diet, including tube feedings. If a prealbumin level check has not been completed, the dietician works with nurses and physicians to obtain the level.

Unit champions consider it a personal affront if a pressure ulcer occurs on a patient under their care. They assume responsibility to assure that staff are fully aware of the protocol, complete chart audits, and directly intervene with staff whose documentation is not compliant with the protocol. In other words, they have integrated the evidence-based practice protocols into their care and demonstrate ownership of outcomes.

Physical therapists are now consulted by nursing staff to perform passive and active range of motion on all bed-bound patients; nurses now consult the clinical nurse specialist for wound care and have involved patients and their families in the assessing to assure that the protocol is followed consistently.

These results are astounding and reflect the integration of care that can result when project planning is carefully completed and the project management follows the plan, allowing for flexibility in responding to circumstances that can arise.

References

Lyder, C. (2003). Pressure ulcer prevention and management. *JAMA, 289*(2), 223–226.
National Pressure Ulcer Advisory Panel, Cuddigan, J., Ayello, E., & Sussman, C. (Eds.). (2001). *Pressure ulcers in America: Prevalence, incidence, and implication for the future.* Reston, VA: NPUAP.

Pressure Ulcer Audit Tool

Please complete a separate form for each pressure ulcer that develops during patient's hospitalization.

Upon completion send to Rigg Curtis.

Nursing unit _____ Admitting diagnosis _____

Audit date _____

Risk factors. Circle each risk factor.

    a. Unstable spine, date cleared _____

    b. Paraplegia

  c. Quadriplegia
  d. Braden < 16
  e. Multisystem failure
  f. Preexisting wound
  g. Complete bed rest
  h. Bowel incontinence
  i. Bladder incontinence
  j. Prealbumin < 18
  k. Diabetic
  l. Emaciated
  m. Obesity
  n. Albumin < 3.5

Patient on a firm surface for a prolonged period (emergency department, surgery, radiology, cardiac cath lab, etc.).

  Y ❑ Length of time _____
  N ❑

Patient's current medication includes:

  a. Paralytics   Y ❑ N ❑
  b. Vasopressors   Y ❑ N ❑
  c. Sedatives   Y ❑ N ❑

Pressure Ulcer Risk Information

  1. Initial skin assessment documented
    on patient data profile.   Y ❑ N ❑
  2. Initial Braden scale risk assessment
    documented on patient data profile. Y ❑ N ❑
  3. Reassessment of Braden scale performed
    and documented every 12 hours.   Y ❑ N ❑

Last Braden score _____   Date _____

Nutrition:

a. Nutrition consultation: Y ❏   N ❏

b. NPO: Y ❏   N ❏

c. Tube feeding Y ❏   N ❏   Meet goal: Y ❏   N ❏

   Date _____

d. Feed self: Y ❏   N ❏

e. TPN: Y ❏   N ❏

f. P.O. intake < 50%: Y ❏   N ❏

Pressure ulcer location _____ Stage _____

What preventive measures were taken?

a. Overlay: Y ❏   N ❏

b. Prealbumin: Y ❏   N ❏

c. Nutritional consultation: Y ❏   N ❏

d. Wound care initiated: Y ❏   N ❏

Action plan: _____

_____

_____

Figure 13-6 Assessment.

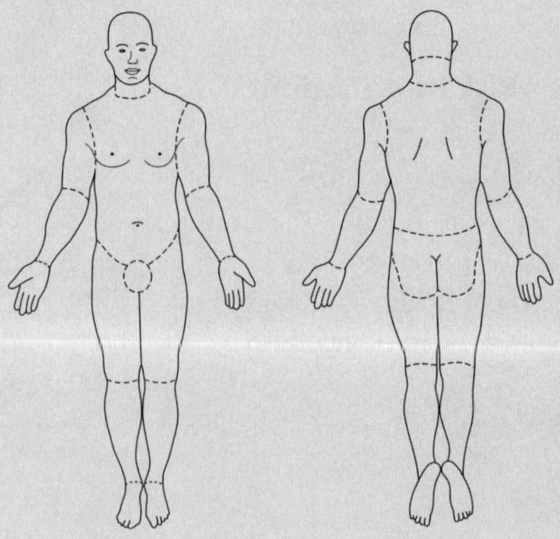

Revision of a Clinical Ladder: A Journey to Professionalism

Valorie Dearmon

Problem Statement

Retaining and recruiting qualified registered nurses can be fostered if a clinical ladder is present. Clinical ladders promote professional development and result in enhanced nurse satisfaction and positive outcomes. This project was aimed at transforming a task-oriented clinical ladder program into a professional practice model at an academic medical healthcare center in the southeastern United States.

Knowledge Gap

To achieve the project aim, framing actions that increased professional autonomy and accountability, dissemination of best practice, professional development promotion, and integration of the program into the performance evaluation system was required.

Team Development and Inclusion/Project Processes

A needs assessment and staff surveys that focused on the current program, processes required to redesign, and staff satisfaction were conducted. A dedicated team was appointed, and through guided direction, a new program, professional advancement for clinical excellence, was proposed to management. The clinical practice program was used as the supporting template and encouraged accountability and professionalism and is based on Benner's 2001 work and the American Nurses Association scope and standards of practice.

Outcomes

The new clinical ladder program included four tiers, and new standards for RN performance evaluation were developed. Consensus was reached that for advancement, a BSN was required. Unexpectedly, economic realities resulted in no resources to implement the new program. Remarkably, the staff unanimously voted to implement the program with or without added compensation. The value of the new program is in the process of being evaluated.

Reference

Benner, P. (2001). *From novice to expert: Excellence and power in clinical nursing practice* (commemorative ed.). Upper Saddle River, NJ: Prentice Hall.

The Development of a Clinical Nurse Leader Residency Program

Paula Miller

Problem Statement

A program being used in healthcare organizations that has an effect on clinical patient care outcomes and nursing satisfaction is the clinical nurse leader (CNL) program. This new nursing role was implemented to support clinical nursing at the bedside and promote evidence-based practice in nursing in the clinical area (American Association of Colleges of Nursing, 2007). The patient care outcomes from the work of the CNLs in these programs are just being identified. Also being identified by these CNLs are their difficulties entering into nursing practice as a pioneering new role in nursing. The project was developed after anecdotal notations from conferences, e-mail lists, and personal communication with practicing CNLs who identified dissatisfaction with the role of immersion experience into nursing practice.

Knowledge Gap/Team Inclusion

Recognizing and using observations and comments as triggers, a needs assessment can be useful for CNLs in identifying and addressing issues. The triggers are identified by the CNLs who are entering practice where a lack of CNL role clarity and delineation from other nursing roles and difficulty in implementing evidence-based practice principles exist within the clinical environment. CNLs identified these difficulties as resulting in a delay in successfully implementing components of the CNL role involving program development and evidence-based practice. This delay in implementing the CNL role could affect the development of quality improvement programs in the clinical environment, which ultimately would affect the delivery of quality nursing care (Bowcutt, Wall, & Goolsby, 2006; Harris, Tornabeni, & Walters 2006).

Nurse residency programs exist for new nurses graduating from professional nursing programs; however, no residency program currently exists for the CNL. The decision to create such a CNL residency program came about to satisfy course requirements; however, the author soon recognized this as an opportunity to work on creating a residency program that would enhance clinical outcomes of the CNL through the timely application of quality care management. This soon became a goal in not only advancing my personal satisfaction as a nurse, but as an opportunity to advance my leadership skills within my organization.

Project Processes

Working within the framework of the American Association of Colleges of Nursing's (AACN) eight essentials of doctoral education for advanced practice nursing (AACN, 2006), work toward developing a clinical nurse leader residency program (CNLRP) was begun. Hence, working to develop a CNLRP involved conceptualizing the issues identified by the CNLs, and identifying methods to resolve these concerns, thereby ensuring an efficient streamlined process for the CNL immersion into clinical practice is guiding the project.

The Iowa model of evidence-based practice to promote quality care (Titler, 2002) guided the CNLRP program development combined with the University of South Alabama's DNP systems improvement model created by Dr. Catherine Dearman and Dr. Linda Roussel (2008). The Johns Hopkins nursing evidence-based practice model and guidelines were chosen to guide the CNL in the implementation of the principles of EBP at the bedside along with the plan, do, study, act (PDSA) method for development of quality process improvements. The program used to guide the overall project planning involved with the CNLRP was the Lewis method of project management (Lewis, 2005). The CNLRP would involve a system change for healthcare organizations, so to assist my leadership skills in dealing with the conflicts that are involved with introducing a change process, the eight-stage process for implementing major change (Kotter, 1996) was selected to guide this transformational change.

Evaluation and Outcomes

As development of the CNLRP began, it was evident that outcomes would be a valuable component in determining the success of this program. Not only would satisfaction of the identified triggers of CNL role (role clarity/delineation and applications of EBP principles) be measured, but the outcomes of program development within nursing practice by the CNL would also need to be part of the evaluation component. Following the Institute of Medicine's six aims for healthcare improvement (safe, effective, efficient, patient-centered, timely, and equitable), an evaluation tool was created to monitor the outcomes of the CNLRP program based on these aims, along with a tool to guide the evaluation of the CNL process improvements.

During the planning stage for the CNLRP, the Lewis (2005) method of project management was used to determine and manage the strategic approach to creating the program. Since the program involved many stakeholders at different levels within different organizational systems, this guide was helpful in directing initial planning and maintaining a consistent approach to problem solving. As the project vision was identified and conceptualized, Titler's Iowa model directed the overall work involved in creating an evidence-based practice change. This involved defining the action plan, forming a team, assembling relevant research, and determining the change process, which are all important elements for consideration in developing a quality improvement program. The Iowa model provided the format to follow and institute an EBP change that identified the gap between current practice (what was going on) and research or evidence available that provided guidelines to practice (what should be) as described by Dontje (2008).

The system change itself was directed using University of South Alabama's system change model, which maintained the focus of quality improvement using an evidence-based program development approach that was sustainable over time and that would affect patient care using various levels of change over a period of time. The University of South Alabama model determined the focus of the project, which involved both a clinical and an organizational focus. The CNLRP's clinical focus involved implementing a patient care improvement program to direct clinical leaders, while the organizational focus involved implementing a system change in the manner in which these leaders were immersed into clinical practice.

As the program development began, the problem was identified, knowledge-focused triggers were collected, and the level of priority for use of a CNLRP within the organization was identified. A team was formed using a facility mentor, an organizational consultant, and faculty members from the University of South Alabama DNP program. As research evidence was collected and evaluated, the amount of relevant research relating to a CNL residency program was limited; however, the research validating the successful outcomes of utilizing nurse residency programs were numerous. Expert opinions in the CNL role development with outcomes to this role were found in peer-reviewed journals and identified based on relevancy to the program.

It became clear after starting the DNP program how the eight essentials of DNP nursing would become applicable in my career. Program and role development at this level went hand in hand and certainly took a higher road as it prepared me at a different level of program development and management. The DNP degree is a new model for nursing education with outcomes just being demonstrated. Within my own experience, the application of critical thinking in program development of a program such as the CNLRP has certainly been enhanced through the application of the principles obtained in the training received from the DNP program.

References

American Association of Colleges of Nursing. (2006). *The essentials of doctoral practice for advanced nursing practice.* Retrieved from http://www.aacn.nche.edu/DNP /index.htm

American Association of Colleges of Nursing. (2007). *White paper on the education and role of the clinical nurse leader.* Retrieved from http://www.aacn.nche.edu /CNLWhitPaper.html

Bowcutt, M., Wall, J., & Goolsby, M. J. (2006). The clinical nurse leader: Promoting patient-centered outcomes. *Nursing Administration Quarterly, 30*(2), 156–161.

Dearman, C., & Roussel, L. (2008). *University of South Alabama, DNP system change model.* Retrieved from http://usaonline.southalabama.edu

Dontje, K. J. (2008). Evidence-based practice: Understanding the process. *Topics in Advanced Practice Nursing eJournal >NONPF Educator's Forum.* Retrieved from http://www.medscape.com/viewarticle/567786_print

Harris, J. L., Tornabeni, J., & Walters, S. E. (2006). The clinical nurse leader: A valued member of the healthcare team. *Journal of Nursing Administration, 36*(10), 446–449.

Kotter, J. P. (1996). *Leading change.* Boston: Harvard Business School Press.

Lewis, J. P. (2005). *Project planning, scheduling and control: A hands-on guide to bringing projects in on time and on budget* (4th ed). New York: McGraw-Hill.

Titler, M. (2002). *National Nursing Practice Network: Iowa model of evidence-based practice to promote quality care introduction.* Retrieved from http://www.nnpnetwork.org /promotion/iowa-model.html

Development of an Administrative Plan to Design and Implement a Shared Governance Model

Gregory S. Eagerton

Problem Statement

Unexpected registered nurse (RN) turnover rates can lead to lower staffing levels and higher nurse-to-patient ratios and impact patient care and safety (Holtom & O'Neill, 2004; Jones & Gates, 2007; Leners, Wilson, Connon, & Fenton, 2006). A major factor that leads to turnover is dissatisfaction with the level of nurse-perceived input in management of work environments. A shared governance model supports nurse involvement at all organizational levels; however, a well-crafted administrative plan promotes successful implementation.

Knowledge Gap

This project was designed to develop an administrative plan as the foundation for implementation of a shared governance model implementation, thus reducing RN turnover.

Project Processes

Guiding the project was a time-specific plan that included objectives, project action(s), required resources, and target completion dates. The project plan and timeline are included in **Table 13-3**.

Table 13-3 DNP Project Plan and Timeline

Objective	Project Action(s)	Required Resources	Target Completion Date
Assess need for change in practice			
1. Review baseline data on registered nurse turnover rates at organization.	1. Gain support of nursing leadership members through education and discussion.	1. Time to teach and discuss concepts of shared governance with nursing leadership members	Month 1
2. Identify survey tool that assesses levels of satisfaction for identified attributes.	2. Identify survey tool that assesses seven attributes.	2. Time to review survey tools	
3. Analyze data from survey.	3. Identify gap analysis process for use by organizations.		
4. Communicate the problem with stakeholders.			
5. Perform gap analysis.			
Link problem with interventions and outcomes			
1. Communicate gap analysis results with stakeholders.	1. Review literature for shared governance educational materials to be used by organizations.	1. Time for review of literature	Month 3
2. Educate stakeholders on concepts of shared governance.	2. Talk with leaders and educators in organizations with shared governance to determine what is used for education.	2. Time to identify organizations with shared governance models and identify those responsible for educating stakeholders about shared governance	

(continues)

Table 13-3 DNP Project Plan and Timeline *(continued)*

Objective	Project Action(s)	Required Resources	Target Completion Date
Synthesize best evidence			
1. Conduct review of literature on shared governance.	1. Continue to review literature on shared governance.	1. Time to review literature	Month 3
2. Identify best model for organization.	2. Discuss best evidence utilized by other organizations.	2. Time with leaders of other organizations to discuss their evidence-based practices	
Design a change in practice			
1. Establish a shared governance steering committee (includes identifying members and charging group with their roles, responsibilities, and accountability).	1. Review literature and establish considerations for membership to steering committee and subcommittees.	1. Time for review of literature	Month 5
	2. Identify from the literature and organizations utilizing shared governance roles and responsibilities of steering committee and subcommittees.	2. Time for interviewing other organizations about their committee and subcommittee structure and teaching materials	
2. Establish subcommittees as needed (may be based upon number and type of attributes being measured and addressed).		3. Time for developing a cost-analysis tool	

3. Educate committee and subcommittees about shared governance.
4. Develop communication and education plan for stakeholders.
5. Conduct cost analyses.
6. Establish mutually agreed-upon goals and timelines for committees and subcommittees.

3. Identify educational materials to use for teaching steering committee, subcommittees, and stakeholders about shared governance principles.
4. Identify best practices for communicating with stakeholders.
5. Develop cost analysis tool.

Implement and evaluate change in practice

1. Establish reasonable timelines.
2. Monitor resource utilization.
3. Measure outcomes.
4. Communicate with stakeholders.

1. Review literature and interview organizations with shared governance about reasonable timelines.
2. Identify outcome measures.

1. Time for literature review and interviews
2. Time for identifying outcome measures

Month 7

(continues)

Table 13-3 CNP Project Plan and Timeline (*continued*)

Objective	Project Action(s)	Required Resources	Target Completion Date
Integrate and maintain a change in practice			
1. Determine scope of pilot, i.e., use on unit as pilot site or use all units during pilot phase? 2. Based on findings of pilot, plan for integration throughout the organization if determined to be best model. 3. Develop monitors to ensure maintenance of new structure.	1. Evaluate tools for monitoring maintenance of changes.	1. Time for literature review and interviews with other organizations successful at maintaining shared governance models	Month 12

Evaluation Methods

The administrative plan's impact will be measured by the degree to which the shared governance model is developed and implemented. The ultimate goal of the project is to decrease turnover of registered nurses; therefore, measuring turnover rates is the primary measurement that will be tracked to measure the effectiveness of a shared governance plan. The baseline data already exist via the recruitment office. Rosswurm and Larrabee's (1999) change model will serve as the framework for the project and guides the development of the administrative plan. Specifically, the components focus on the following.

- Assess need for change in practice.
- Link problem with interventions and outcomes.
- Synthesize best evidence.
- Design a change in practice.
- Implement and evaluate change in practice.
- Integrate and maintain change in practice.

Planned Processes and Anticipated Outcomes

Outcomes will be in the form of an administrative plan set of tools that can be utilized as an organization prepares to implement shared governance. The plan and tools can be used for data collection and analysis, providing staff education, identifying and using a shared governance steering committee, and as a means by which the changes made through shared governance can be sustained.

References

Holtom, B. C., & O'Neill, B. S. (2004). Job embeddedness: A theoretical foundation for developing a comprehensive nurse retention plan. *Journal of Nursing Administration, 34*(5), 216–227.

Jones, C. B., & Gates, M. (2007). The costs and benefits of nurse turnover: A business case for nurse retention. *Online Journal of Issues in Nursing, 12*(3), Retrieved from www.cinahl.com/cgi-bin/refsvc?jid=1331&aacmp=2009867880

Leners, D., Wilson, V., Connor, P., & Fenton, J. (2006). Mentorship: Increasing retention probabilities. *Journal of Nursing Management, 14*(8), 652–654.

Rosswurm, M. A., & Larrabee, J. H. (1999). A model for change to evidence-based practice. *Image Journal of Nursing Scholarship, 31*(4), 317–322.

Improving Cardiovascular Disease Risk Factors in Overweight and Obese Women

An Intervention Promoting a Healthy Lifestyle Using the New Leaf Model

Robin Lawson

Problem Statement

Obesity is one of the most prevalent health concerns in our society, and Alabama is ranked as the one of the fattest states in the nation. In comparison to other states, Alabama deaths due to heart disease, stroke, and diabetes (all conditions associated with diabetes) are ranked as some of the highest. The people in the counties in the southernmost third of Alabama are more likely to be at risk. Health disparities that place individuals at greater risk include low socioeconomic status, uninsured status, and low literacy rates. Uninsured women are especially vulnerable to cardiovascular disease (CVD) and other chronic illnesses. Risk factors associated with the prevalence of CVD in women typically include body mass index ≥ 30, waist circumference ≥ 35 inches, fasting glucose ≥ 100, and systolic blood pressure ≥ 130 or diastolic blood pressure ≥ 85. An estimated 1,600 patients at the project site, a healthcare clinic for uninsured individuals in Mobile, Alabama, are considered obese. Approximately two thirds of the patients are women. A needs assessment of the clinic revealed that a structured method of providing adequate and consistent educational information and services for the prevention and treatment of obesity was not in place. Evidence supports a therapeutic lifestyle approach with a healthy diet and increased physical activity.

Knowledge Gap and Team Inclusion

The aims of the project were to improve CVD risk factors in overweight or obese low-income, uninsured women at the clinic and to propose a protocol for identifying at-risk women through the clinic who could be targeted for inclusion in a CVD risk reduction program. The literature reviewed for this project was found to be of high-grade quality and of particular relevance to the vulnerable population of overweight and obese, low-income women at risk for developing CVD. The innovative strategy selected to improve patient outcomes was *A New Leaf . . . Choices for Healthy Living,* the structured evidence-based assessment and counseling intervention component of the Well-Integrated Screening and Evaluation for Women Across the Nation program that was developed by the Centers for Disease Control and Prevention and first administered by the North Carolina Department of Public Health and Human Services. Several conceptual and theoretical frameworks were used to guide the project. Such frameworks included the IOM, the ace star model of knowledge transformation, and the socioecological model of health promotion. Major project supporters and collaborative partners included the Alabama Department of Public Health Office of Women's Health, the Alabama Cooperative Extension Agency, and the clinic's medical director.

Project Processes and Evaluation Methods

Prior to implementation, institutional review board approval was obtained. After participants signed a consent form, a baseline screening was done to assess for risk factors and conditions requiring medical clearance. At week 1, participants had physical measurements (i.e., weight, body mass index, waist circumference, blood pressure, and blood glucose) taken and completed a pretest that addressed the types of foods they ate, their physical activity levels, and their self-confidence levels. The program included a total of 10 one-hour sessions held over a three-month time period. At week 12, participants completed a posttest that was identical to the pretest and had their final physical measurements taken. These measures comprised the quantitative component of the project. Privacy and confidentiality were maintained, and protocols ensuring reliability and validity of the measures were followed. Qualitative data obtained from additional activities added depth and detail to the quantitative findings. Such activities included participant focus group discussions, administrator/healthcare provider focus group discussions, and observation note recordings.

Four basic outcomes of the project were expected. The first expected outcome was that there would be increased obesity awareness among participants. The second expected outcome was that there would be a reduction in participant CVD risk factors. The third expected outcome was that the overall program would be effective. The fourth expected outcome was that the clinic would adopt the protocol for identifying at-risk women.

Outcomes

Findings revealed that all of project specified were met and in accordance with the expected outcomes. Detailed results of the objectives were: (1) A total of 37 participants were enrolled in the project at week 1, and 21 remained enrolled at week 12. (2) All participants enrolled at week 1 were surveyed as to how many times they ate certain foods, how often they performed particular physical activities in an average day, and their confidence levels. (3) Educational sessions using the new leaf model that focused on nutrition or physical activity were held weekly during the first 8 weeks and biweekly during the last month. Baseline screenings and assessments were done. (4a) Four of the six participants' physical measurements (i.e., weight, body mass index, waist circumference, and systolic blood pressure) showed statistically significant improvements. Many of the participants' self-reported items addressing types of food eaten, physical activity, and confidence levels also showed statistically significant improvements. The evaluation was based on a comparison of the means for week 1 and week 12. (4b) An in-depth qualitative assessment using additional measures of effectiveness derived from group discussion key concepts and observation notes of project processes resulted in identification of important strengths and weaknesses that provided insight into the development of a protocol for identifying at-risk women at the clinic for inclusion in and sustainability of a CVD risk reduction program. (5) The final objective of proposing a protocol for identifying female patients at risk for CVD through the clinic was accomplished. The protocol included not only use of a risk assessment tool for identifying patients at risk, but also a method for keeping track of those patients identified for inclusion in a CVD risk reduction program. Subsequently, the protocol was adopted by the clinic.

In summary, obesity and obesity-related health problems such as CVD are major health issues, and effective methods aimed at reducing these problems are necessary. An assessment revealed the need to improve the process of providing appropriate care to overweight and obese women at the project site. The literature review provided valuable insight as to the most effective way to approach the problem. The project produced a significant reduction in CVD risk factors in overweight and obese women at the project site over a 3-month period by using an effective, patient-centered approach. An evaluation of the overall project, including processes, further validated its effectiveness. Adoption of the protocol by the clinic to identify at-risk women for inclusion in a CVD risk reduction program will help others reduce their risks. Additional projects incorporating lifestyle changes such as healthy diet and increased physical activity, tracking lipids, and/or lowering stress as a means to reduce CVD risk factors are recommended.

Suggested Readings

Alabama Department of Public Health. (2005). *Alabama obesity task force strategic plan for the prevention and control of overweight and obesity in Alabama.* Retrieved from http://www.adph.org/NUTRITION/assets/ObesityPlan.pdf

Alabama Department of Public Health. (2006). *Risk of overweight and obesity in Alabama: Results from the Behavioral Risk Factor Surveillance System, Alabama 2004.* Retrieved from http://www.adph.org/obesity/assets/Obesitybycounty2007.1.05.10.pdf

Centers for Disease Control and Prevention. (2008). *Alabama: Burden of chronic diseases.* Retrieved from http://www.cdc.gov/chronicdisease/states/pdf/alabama.pdf

Centers for Disease Control and Prevention. (2009). *Wisewoman—Preventing disease among women most in need: At a glance 2009.* Retrieved from http://www.cdc.gov /chronicdisease/resources/publications/AAG/wisewoman.htm

Galassi, A., Reynolds, K., & Jiang, H. (2006). Metabolic syndrome and risk of cardiovascular disease: A meta-analysis. *The American Journal of Medicine, 119*(10), 812–819.

Gami, A. S., Witt, B. J., Howard, D. E., Erwin, P. J., Gami, L. A., Somers, V. K., et al. (2007). Metabolic syndrome and risk of incident cardiovascular events and death. *Journal of the American College of Cardiology, 49*(4), 403–414.

Grundy, S. M., Cleeman, J. I., Daniels, S. R., Donato, K. A., Eckel, R. H., Franklin, B. A., et al. (2005). Diagnosis and management of the metabolic syndrome. American Heart Association/National Heart, Lung, and Blood Institute scientific statement and executive summary. *Circulation Journal of the American Heart Association, 112,* 2735–2752. Retrieved from http://circ.ahajournals.org/cgi/reprint/112/17/2735

Lorenzo, C., Williams, K., Hunt, K. J., & Haffner, S. M. (2007). The National Cholesterol Education Program—Adult Treatment Panel III, International Diabetes Federation, and World Health Organization definitions of the metabolic syndrome as predictors of incident cardiovascular disease and diabetes. *Diabetes Care, 30*(1), 8–13. Retrieved from http://care.diabetesjournals.org/content/30/1/8.full.pdf+html

Mosca, L., Banka, C. L., Benjamin, E. J., Berra, K., Bushnell, C., & Dolor, R. J. (2007). AHA guideline. Evidence-based guidelines for cardiovascular disease prevention: 2007 update. *Journal of the American College of Cardiology, 49*(11), 1230–1250.

Trust for America's Health. (2009). *New report finds Alabama has 2nd highest percent of obese adults and 6th highest percent of obese and overweight children in the U.S.* Retrieved from http://healthyamericans.org/reports/obesity2009/release .php?stateid=AL

University of North Carolina at Chapel Hill Health Promotion and Disease Prevention. (n.d.). *A new leaf... Choices for healthy living.* Retrieved from http://www.hpdp.unc .edu/WISEWOMAN/newleaf.htm

U.S. Department of Health and Human Services and U.S. Department of Agriculture. (2005). *Dietary guidelines for Americans, 2005* (6th ed.). Retrieved from http://www .health.gov/DietaryGuidelines/dga2005/document/default.htm

FOURTEEN

Voices From the Field: Best Project Plans From Practice

■ Catherine Dearman, Linda Roussel, and
Lonnie K. Williams

■ Learning Objectives

1. Analyze project exemplars across practice settings from practice and administrative experts.
2. Discuss the importance of projects that add value to patient care and systems outcomes.

> "Be the change you wish to see in the world."
>
> —Gandhi

Introduction

Project management is an ongoing process. Introduced into graduate curricula, students learn the didactics of putting a project together including doing a needs assessment, using the best evidence to support credible interventions, and using metrics that matter in the implementation and **evaluation** of outcomes. This chapter provides exemplars from seasoned practitioners on projects that have demonstrated positive outcomes evidenced by increased efficiency, efficacy, and patient-centered care.

Key Terms

Change

Evaluation

Innovation

Value

Roles

Communicator

Decision maker

Designer

Educator

Leader

Professional Values

Evidence-based practice

Integrity

Quality

Core Competencies

Anticipation

Communication

Coordination

Design

Project management

Resource management

Application of the Clinical Nurse Leader Role in the Outpatient Clinical Setting

Alicia Drew

Problem Statement

The clinical nurse leader (CNL) role as a master's-prepared nurse generalist has broad application to multiple care settings. The literature is sparse on application of the CNL in the outpatient setting, with case studies, examples, and comments most often referring to the role in the acute care setting.

However, according to the Kaiser Family Foundation (2009), only 31% of total healthcare spending ($2.2 trillion) in 2007 was for hospital-based care. Economic factors and changing reimbursement structure will likely further increase the amount of care provided in outpatient settings.

The American Association of Colleges of Nursing (2007) states the CNL role not only applies to acute care, but can provide leadership in all aspects of the healthcare system. CNL educational preparation provides a broad base of knowledge to draw upon when functioning in the outpatient setting, which may include program development and administration or population-specific application such as an oncology nurse navigator.

The CNL can effectively and efficiently function in the outpatient setting, which often requires one to multitask duties and responsibilities. Application of the American Association of Colleges of Nursing CNL core competencies and the health professions core competencies identified by the Institute of Medicine, which include patient-centered care, interdisciplinary teams, evidence-based practice, quality improvement, and informatics, were used to structure the project (Finkelman & Kenner, 2009).

Gap in Knowledge Addressed by the Project

An analysis of the current status of health care today indicated that only 31% of total healthcare spending ($2.2 trillion) in 2007 was for hospital-based care (Kaiser Family Foundation, 2009); approximately 902 million physician office visits occurred in 2006 (Cherry, Hing, Woodwell & Rechtsteiner, 2008); an estimated 102.2 million hospital outpatient department visits occurred in 2006 (Hing, Hall, & Xu, 2008); approximately 119.2 million emergency department visits occurred in 2006 (Pitts, Niska, Xu, & Burt, 2008), and approximately 34.9 million hospital discharges (excluding newborns) occurred in 2006 (DeFrances, Lucas, Buie, & Golosinskiy, 2008).

Changes in care delivery and reimbursement structure, as well as economic factors, will likely further increase the amount of care provided in outpatient settings. The CNL is prepared to respond to increasing and changing demands of today's outpatient care environment. The project was designed to address the role development in the outpatient setting.

Team Development

Working with the breast cancer clinic team, the CNL coordinated screenings, along with selected services and outreach education in the community.

Process Management

The CNL assessed the environment of an outpatient breast cancer clinic and found a need to identify patients at risk for breast cancer, promoting appropriate screening, connecting the patient to appropriate services, and providing ongoing breast cancer awareness education to the community.

As a part of this project, the CNL continually evaluated current outcomes measures and suggested new outcomes measures to account for necessary care changes such as decreasing the number of days from suspicious findings to biopsy, and the frequency of postprocedure infection. In the outpatient setting, the role of the CNL with providers is to assure that providers stay informed of emerging research and technologies; policies, procedures, and care are based on the latest evidence and patient preference; and develop clinical protocols or checklists for various groups of patients with commonality (for example, all at high genetic risk for breast cancer; all with a new diagnosis of cancer).

The role of the CNL with patients is to assure that the patient has information to make informed decisions; assure that support services (support groups, social services, financial assistance, etc.) are accessed and available; evaluate individuals at risk related to new diagnoses and chronic/preexisting conditions; evaluate risks commonly associated with groups (for example, increased risk of infection and potential decreased nutritional status of patients receiving chemotherapy); use a variety of methods to provide education about diagnosis, treatment, medications, etc.; and continually assess needs as patients progress through the care continuum.

In order to accomplish these ambitious goals, the CNL participated and encouraged continuing education; promoted evidence-based practice (EBP) across the entire multidisciplinary healthcare team; and assessed information-sharing capabilities across the interdisciplinary team and facilitated improvement.

Evaluation Methods

Evaluation methods included ongoing staff and patient feedback on breast cancer screenings and community education. As a part of this project, the CNL continually evaluated current outcomes measures and suggested new outcomes measures to account for necessary care changes such as decreasing the number of days from suspicious findings to biopsy.

Outcomes With Impact

The breast care screening project continues via programs within cancer care for patients in the community.

References

American Association of Colleges of Nursing. (2007). *White paper on the education and role of the clinical nurse leader.* Retrieved from http://aacn.nche.edu/Publications/WhitePapers/ClinicalNurseLeader07.pdf

Cherry, D. K., Hing, E., Woodwell, D. A., & Rechtsteiner, E. A. (2008). *National ambulatory medical care survey: 2006 summary* (National Health Statistics Reports No. 3, August 6). Retrieved from http://www.cdc.gov/nchs/data/nhsr/nhsr003.pdf

DeFrances, C. J., Lucas, C. A., Buie, V. C., & Golosinskiy, A. (2008). *2006 national hospital discharge survey* (National Health Statistics Reports No. 5, July 30). Retrieved from http://www.cdc.gov/nchs/data/nhsr/nhsr005.pdf

Finkelman, A., & Kenner, C. (2010). *Professional nursing concepts: Competencies for quality leadership.* Sudbury, MA: Jones and Bartlett.

Hing, E., Hall, M. J., & Xu, J. (2008). *National hospital ambulatory medical care survey: 2006 outpatient department summary* (National Health Statistics Reports No. 4, August 6, 2008). Retrieved from http://www.cdc.gov/nchs/data/nhsr/nhsr004.pdf

Kaiser Family Foundation. (2009). *U.S. health care costs: Background brief.* Retrieved from http://www.kaiseredu.org/topics_im.asp?id=358&imID=1&parentID=61

Pitts, S. R., Niska, R. W., Xu, J., & Burt, C. W. (2008). *National hospital ambulatory medicalcare survey: 2006 emergency department summary* (National Health Statistics Reports No. 7, August 6). Retrieved from http://www/cdc/gov/nchs/data/nhsr/nhsr007.pdf

The Clinical Nurse Leader and Transforming Care at the Bedside: A Winning Combination

Becky Pomrenke

Problem Statement

The University of South Alabama Medical Center (USAMC) identified quality issues with patient care and meeting national guidelines. As a safety net facility, the USAMC provides care to the underinsured and uninsured at a greater percentage than other facilities in the area, including 39% who self-pay, 15% who receive Medicare benefits, and 15% who receive Medicaid benefits. The case mix index of 2.3 placed USAMC at 44th in the nation. National benchmarking values were compared to the outcomes of the USAMC, and variances were identified. As a direct result, the facility embarked on a project to improve the quality and safety of patient care delivered. As a part of participating in the Robert Wood Johnson Foundation's Transforming Care at the Bedside project, the USAMC nursing and hospital administrators selected the sixth floor, a 35-bed trauma, orthopedics, and general surgery unit as the test site, and the fifth floor as the control unit. The sixth floor had an average daily census of 35, an average of 96 patient admissions per month, and an average of 960 patient days per month. Twenty-seven full-time and three part-time RNs comprised the staffing. Baseline data reflected a direct care average of 58.2%, which was 6.3% higher than the national mean. **Value-**added care averaged 60% at the beginning of the project and 70% at the end, a gain of 10%, placing the USAMC at 11% higher than the national average.

Gap in Knowledge Addressed by the Project

This academic health center was experiencing a pressure ulcer rate of 7.8%, higher than the national mean of 7%; and less than satisfactory patient satisfaction and urinary catheter infection rates. The project was designed to monitor the work of the RN staff and measure the amount of time spent on various duties, e.g., documentation, hunting and gathering supplies, etc.

Team Development

The project was directed by the CNL on the unit. Other members of the team included the unit manager of sixth floor, the unit manager of the fifth floor, the unit-based educator on both units, and a member of the college of nursing faculty who is skilled in quality and safety processes.

Process Management

The needs assessment had already been performed, so the project director completed a gap and workflow analysis to compare baseline status on the unit to best practices. The CNL implemented a tracking system using a personal data assistant (PDA) to collect data. Each nurse had a PDA, and when the alarm went off, he or she documented what he or she was doing immediately previous to the alarm and what he or she planned to do next. The CNL maintained an **innovation** log and monthly data sheets to track activities and monitor for achievement of benchmarks. The innovation log and monthly data sheets were essential to providing a baseline data on call light frequency, staff overtime in hours and in dollars, and incidences of never events such as urinary tract infections and pressure ulcers.

The PDA data was sent electronically to become a part of the National Benchmarking Project that measures direct and value-added care.

Evaluation Methods

Evaluation methods included the PDA data set, patient satisfaction data, as well as the never events.

Outcomes With Impact

Since October of 2007, there have been no patient falls with harm, a presumed impact of the hourly rounding intervention. In association with bedside reporting, the amount of time required for each RN to see all of his or her patients went from 90 minutes to 30 minutes at the beginning of each shift. Over the same time frame, the rate of pressure ulcers dropped from 2% to less than 1% and no pressure ulcers were found to be greater than stage 2 on evaluation. The implementation of pain boards (white boards placed in patient rooms to document administration of pain medications) resulted in greater patient and nurse satisfaction as well as better pain control; after the successful trial period, this innovation was spread to the all medical surgical units throughout the facility. The CNL is the go-to person for staff related to transforming care at the bedside. The staff and patients are energized and have an active voice in **change**. The CNL assists the staff in finding and implementing innovations in response to need and presents the innovations and outcomes associated to administrators on behalf of the staff.

References

Kemski, A. (2002). Market forces, cost assumptions, and nurse supply: Considerations in determining appropriate nurse to patient ratios in general acute care hospitals R-37-01, SEIU Nurse Alliance, December, as cited in *The costs and benefits of safe staffing ratios, fact sheet 2004*, The Department for Professional Employees, AFL=CIO. Retrieved from www.dpeaflcio.org/policy/factsheets/fs_2004_staffratio.htm#notes

Lavizzo-Mourey, R., & Berwick, D. M. (2009, November). A special supplement to the *American Journal of Nursing* on transforming care at the bedside: Paving the way for change. Foreword: Nursing Transforming Care. *American Journal of Nursing*, Suppl. *109*(11), p. 3.

Getting to the Core of Opportunity: Using Operational Levels of Control to Improve and Sustain Compliance

Carol J. Ratcliffe

Problem Statement

The Centers for Medicare and Medicaid Services and The Joint Commission require that organizations abstract and submit data on multiple national hospital quality measures. Historically, the pneumonia core measure has been a challenge for many hospitals. Agreement to and required use of a standardized order set, antibiotic selection, antibiotic timing, blood cultures prior to the administration of antibiotics, and the administration of vaccines have presented the greatest challenge. Vaccine administration has been the most difficult challenge of all. The author's organization spent 2 years in a focused effort to improve compliance with the pneumonia core measures. Strategies to improve compliance have focused on feedforward, concurrent, and feedback control across administrative, financial, and quality dimensions.

Gap in Knowledge Addressed by the Project

The author's organizational strategic plan includes specific and concise strategies to improve quality and patient outcomes. Due to the identified opportunities associated with the pneumonia core measures, the organization committed to hiring an outcomes manager to help improve processes and monitor patients with pneumonia concurrently during their hospital stay. This nurse executive was the designated leader for the initiative. This was the beginning of a focused effort to improve compliance with this measure set.

Team Development

The nurse executive formed a multidisciplinary team that included physicians represented by a pulmonologist, a hospitalist, and emergency medicine, nursing, respiratory, quality, pharmacy, and nursing education. This team began by reviewing the core measures for pneumonia, the abstraction definitions, data for the past year by indicator, route of admission (direct admit versus emergency department admission), and by physician. The team also reviewed best practice evidence and compared it to current practice. This plan was inclusive of, but not limited to the establishment of a multidisciplinary team and the recruitment of a pneumonia outcomes manager. The nurse executive served as the leader and facilitator of this team, which heightened the level of commitment by the organization to improve compliance.

Process Management

Through planned development, the organization established administrative, financial, and quality controls to ensure that actions were hardwired in the three phases of organizational control—feedforward, concurrent, and feedback. Through these processes, the organization monitored progress, evaluated deviations from expectations, and developed action plans based on results

(Barnat, n.d.). Following the formation of the team, several initial action steps were identified. These included the need to understand the abstraction guidelines for the measures, review current practices, review data by admission status (direct admit versus emergency department), and identify opportunities. Open dialogue began with the medical staff establishing the foundation for performance improvement through both their department committee meetings and written correspondence. Former practice was compared to evidence-based literature and the core measures, resulting in the development of a pneumonia practice guideline. This included interventions necessary by both the medical staff and nursing associates. Identification triggers were placed in Horizon Enterprise Visibility, which is an information technology system used to manage patient throughput, facilitate communication of orders, identify special needs or risks for patients, and identify patient location.

Administrative: Administrative control facilitates the monitoring of organizational activities based on standard plans and action steps. Through this process, organizations identify strategy, important data elements, and control metrics that will enable success in process implementation and overall outcomes (Daft, 2003). In fiscal year 2008, the organization identified opportunity for improvement related to the pneumonia core measure. As a mechanism to invest the necessary resources to enhance compliance with the measures, the leadership team included the pneumonia core measure as a strategic initiative. For example, the Centers for Medicare and Medicaid Services (CMS) require hospitals to report data on core measures adopted by the Hospital Quality Alliance. This reporting process is a component of a tiered point system linked to reimbursement for Medicare and other commercial payers. The organization is required to abstract and report data on a monthly basis to QNet via an approved CMS database. Hospitals that do not report receive a 2% reduction in their annual payment update by Medicare (QualityNet, n.d.). The pneumonia core measure results are publicly reported and available on the Hospital Compare website. This report compares hospitals to local facilities, the state, and national averages. Public accessibility to data has created a sense of urgency within organizations. Public reporting enables consumers to make decisions based on outcomes and hospital performance. If outcomes are poor compared to others in the market, patient utilization of the organization could be negatively impacted resulting in decreased revenues. Continuous review and revision of processes are necessary to improve outcomes, thus improving data available to the public. The Centers for Medicare and Medicaid are developing a value-based payment structure that will encompass a plan to reimburse hospitals based on performance. When this is developed, specific financial metrics can be established for this core measure. The nurse executive's organization has implemented several quality controls in order to enhance compliance with the pneumonia core measures. These controls have included mandatory staff education on the pneumonia core measures and integration of core measure education into new nurse orientation and distribution of pocket cards. **Exhibit 14-1** illustrates the project controls.

Exhibit 14-1

Operational Controls for the Pneumonia Core Measures

	Feedforward	Concurrent	Feedback
Administrative	Strategic initiative	Practice guideline for pneumonia	Balanced scorecard
	Recruit pneumonia outcomes manager	Monthly pneumonia team meetings	
	Communication letters to physicians	Patient identified in Horizon Enterprise Visibility	
	Pneumonia team action plan	Daily review of charts by nurse manager	
	Team led by vice president	Positive redirection	
		Discharge triggers for vaccines	

(continues)

Exhibit 14-1 *(continued)*

Operational Controls for the Pneumonia Core Measures

	Feedforward	Concurrent	Feedback
Financial	Submission of data to QNet	Revision of processes	Data publicly reported/ Hospital Compare website Balanced scorecard
Quality	Mandatory staff education	Rounds by pneumonia outcomes manager	Control charts
	Core measure education integrated into new nurse orientation	Core measures added to the handoff communication tool	Balanced scorecard
	Pneumonia order set	Vaccines placed in the Pyxis medication dispensing system	Opportunities identified/ appealed
	Vaccine assessment tool/order	Vaccine sticker for front of chart Discharge timeout process	

Evaluation Methods

Chart reviews occur daily by members of nursing leadership to assess for vaccine compliance, which has been the greatest opportunity for improvement. Positive redirection, the organization's method used to change behavior, has been initiated as appropriate. Associate discipline can transition from a coaching to a decision-making leave and is dependent upon an individual's progression in the disciplinary process. Discharge triggers for vaccines were initiated as an additional measure to remind nurses to give vaccines ordered prior to discharge. Lastly, the balanced scorecard was reviewed monthly providing a quick visualization of overall performance. The scorecard enables the linkage between "long-term strategy and short-term actions" (Kaplan & Norton, 2007, p. 152). The balanced scorecard addresses the following perspectives: "translating the vision," "communicating and linking," "business planning," and "feedback and learning" (Kaplan & Norton, 2007, p. 152). The balanced scorecard is used by the organization to depict performance compared to goals. This provides a quick view of overall performance and facilitates the necessary discussion and review of data (control charts) and other findings to determine why and what is causing the deviations from the plan. The nurse executive's organization does not have computerized clinical documentation systems in the emergency department or acute care nursing, necessitating numerous manual processes for concurrent chart audits and control. Bureaucratic measures of control have been dominant in the administrative interventions for this improvement initiative, especially related to nursing compliance. Although the physicians support organizational initiatives to improve patient outcomes and compliance, they are very hesitant to implement the mandatory use of order sets. This facilitates decentralized control to a certain degree, creating opportunities for improvement with some physicians. Use of a mandatory order set would minimize variations in practice. There are 10 measures that are a part of the pneumonia core measure collected and reported to QNet.

Feedforward. Feedforward control is used in anticipation of problems. It is used in an attempt to prevent inappropriate occurrences on the front end. With feedforward, inputs into the organization are the focus, such as human resources. Through this mechanism of control, the organization wants to make sure that it has quality investments up front (Barnat, n.d.; Daft, 2003). The feedforward controls used in this initiative were the following:

- Pneumonia core measure as a strategic initiative
- Recruitment of an outcomes manager

- Communication to physicians
- Formation of a multidisciplinary team and development of an action plan
- Team led by the vice president of patient care services
- Submission of data to QNet
- Mandatory staff education and distribution of pocket cards
- Core measure education integrated into new nurse orientation
- Development of a pneumonia order set
- Use of a vaccine assessment tool and order

Concurrent. Concurrent control is used to ensure that associate actions and interventions are consistent with established standards. Associates will work with others within the organization to revise processes when current ones are not working in order to achieve the intended outcome. This mechanism of control is also referred to as screening control. It monitors real-time activities (Barnat, n.d.; Daft, 2003). The concurrent controls used in this initiative were:

- Establishment of a practice guideline
- Monthly team meetings inclusive of compliance review, process revision, and implementation planning
- Patient identification in Horizon Enterprise Visibility
- Daily chart reviews by the nurse manager
- Use of discharge triggers for vaccines
- Concurrent rounds by the outcomes manager
- Addition of core measures to the handoff communication tool
- Vaccines placed in the Pyxis medication dispensing system for easy access
- Vaccine stickers placed on the front of the chart as a reminder to administer vaccines prior to discharge
- Implementation of a discharge timeout process

Feedback. Feedback control focuses on the quality or outcome of a process. With feedback, outputs of an organization are the focus. This mechanism of control allows an organization to know if its performance is meeting expectations. Feedback can also be used when feedforward and concurrent are too great of an expense to an organization. The feedback phase tells management if their plan was effective. One barrier associated with this phase relates to timeliness of information to management for decision making and revisions to processes (Barnat, n.d.; Daft, 2003). The feedback controls used in this initiative included the balanced scorecard, public reported data on the Hospital Compare website, use of control charts, and opportunities for improvement identified through monthly abstractions analyzed by the patient care unit, by physician, and by nurse. These processes helped to identify trends that needed to be addressed.

Outcomes With Impact

The organization has been very successful in improving compliance through the categories and phases of control described by this nurse executive. Through the concurrent review processes, there has been a continued increase in all measures, with the greatest occurring in vaccine administration. Pneumococcal vaccinations improved from a low of 37.5% to 90% and influenza vaccinations from a low of 66.67% to a high of 100%. Following extensive discussions and review of best practices, the medical staff now allows nurses to administer vaccines based on criteria without an additional physician order prior to discharge. This was a milestone achievement for the pneumonia team. Collaboration between nursing and pharmacy facilitated the transition to single-dosage vaccines and placement at the unit level minimizing delays in administration and missed doses at discharge. The pneumonia core measure composite score improved by 10%. A pneumonia order set was developed by the multidisciplinary team and approved by both the pharmacy and therapeutics committee and the medical executive committee. A vaccine assessment and order tool was developed to serve a dual purpose—patient assessment for vaccine based on approved criteria and as a physician order. The pneumonia outcomes manager rounds daily, reviewing medical records concurrently and interacting with both nursing associates and physicians. In order to enhance communication among caregivers, core measures were added to the tool used to facilitate handoff communication among nursing associates. Vaccines were made available in single-dose injections and placed at the unit level in the Pyxis medication dispensing system. Stickers were placed on the front of the medical record to serve as an additional prompt to staff related to vaccine administration prior to discharge. Control charts were developed for each measure and enable the organization to differ between common cause variation and special cause variation. The multidisciplinary team meets monthly to review control charts and opportunities for improvement by patient care unit, physician, and nursing associate. The order set has been revised to include up-to-date antibiotics guided by the literature and evidence-based practice. Clarity to antibiotic selection has also enhanced compliance to the drug treatment regimen. Although the author's organization has had continued improvement and success associated with the pneumonia core measures, the action plan continues to be revised and updated to capture opportunities to improve patient outcomes and overall hospital performance.

References

Barnat, R. (n.d.). *The evaluation and control of organizational strategy*. Retrieved from http://strategic-control.24xls.com

Daft, R. (2003). *Management* (6th ed.). Mason, OH: Thomson Learning.

Kaplan, R. S., & Norton, D. P. (2007). Using the balanced scorecard as a strategic management system. *Harvard Business Review*, 150–161.

QualityNet. (n.d.). *Reporting hospital quality data for annual payment update*. Retrieved from http://www.qualitynet.org/dcs/ContentServer?c=Page&pagename=QnetPublic%2FPage%2FQnetTier2&cid=1138115987129

Integrating Evidence-Based Practice Into a Veterans Administration Hospital System

Traci Solt

Problem Statement

Evidence based practice (EBP) is the integration of research findings, the best clinical evidence, and examination of a patient's unique values and circumstances to determine nursing care (Polit & Beck, 2008). The lengthy process of applying research at the bedside highlights the urgency for nurses to implement

EBP in everyday patient care. Integration of EBP will encourage practitioners to assess current and past research, clinical guidelines, and other resources to locate and review applicable literature while differentiating between high-quality and low-quality findings. Hardwiring EBP in healthcare facilities will promote quality, cost-effective health care and promote professionalism in nursing practice. Successful program management requires conscientious planning, careful implementation, and thorough evaluation of the process. Implementing new ideas requires change. New programs rolled out without meticulous planning will result in a painful experience.

Gap in Knowledge Addressed by the Project

An agreement was reached at the hospital system that a need existed to improve knowledge, understanding, and use of nurse-driven EBP. During the course of the project, we encountered numerous challenges, won some victories, and gained knowledge along the way.

Team Development

Team members consisted of volunteers who were interested in improving nursing practice and were committed to excellence. The majority of the team consisted of the nursing education department. Because leadership support is essential to successful project implementation, an associate nurse executive was chosen as the goal champion. Once the team was formed and the goal champion chosen, the next step was to agree on objectives required to reach the destination or goal. Our system also had a nursing clinical practice (NCP) committee. This group reviewed and made recommendations related to clinical nursing practice procedures. Building on this information, we built a plan to include and enhance the existing resources.

Process Management

The first step of the project was to define the goal and to determine the current state. Consensus was reached that our target goal was to implement EBP in our hospital system. Investigation began to identify existing efforts related to EBP. Our facility had a loosely run nursing journal club and nursing grand rounds. These activities occurred on alternating months. Both the club meetings and grand rounds were well attended and included participation from bedside nursing, nurse managers, advanced practice nurses, quality management nurses, and executive nursing leadership.

Project planning requires a structured guide similar to a GPS one would use for a cross-country trip. A plan of action and milestones (POA and M) identify goals, assign tasks, and define the measures of completion. Without a clear definition of the goal, it is doubtful the project will reach its destination.

We developed a plan of action and milestones (POA and M) (**Exhibit 14-2**) to lead us on our journey, just as a road map would. Defining our goal and development of a goal statement was the first step in the process to implement EBP. The goal of our project was to implement and increase use of evidence-based practice (EBP) within the Veterans Affairs Gulf Coast Veterans Health Care System nursing.

Once the destination is selected, it is imperative to select a goal champion and identify team members. Without leadership's support and assignment of tasks to team members, projects are confusing and filled with unnecessary obstacles. Confusion related to project goals and objectives can lead to inaccurate and incomplete results that require rework (Roussel, Swansburg, & Swansburg, 2006). Objectives must be clearly written and understood by all members on the project team. Without implicit direction, the risk of rework exists. Rework adds time to a project and leads to decreased morale and unmotivated team members.

We held a meeting to construct our POA and M. We conducted a formal team meeting to generate the objectives. Utilizing the structure of our POA and M, we identified objectives and assigned responsibilities to specific team members. After the objectives were identified, a team was formed and determined it was equally important to define how an objective was attained.

The structure of the POA and M demands that the team state the exact measure of effectiveness. This step is vital to ensure all team members are on the same page. If participants are unclear of the direction and who is required to complete the task, projects will move slowly.

Exhibit 14-2

Projected Plan to Implement and Hardwire EBP at Veterans Affairs Gulf Coast Veterans Healthcare System (VAGCVHCS): Plan of Action and Milestones

Goal: Hardwire use of evidence-based practice (EBP) within the VAGCVHCS nursing.

Goal statement: By March 2011, VAGCVHCS will implement EBP across the continuum in nursing services.

Goal champion: Employee 1
Team members:

Service chief approval date: January 2009

Goal completion date: Pending

Objectives	Action Item	Action Leader/ Start Date	Completion Date	Measure of Effectiveness	Comments
Provide introduction to EBP for VAGCVHCS nursing staff.	Provide introductory overview of EBP using a mock trial approach.	Employee	May 2009—outpatient clinics (45 participants); September 2009—20 participants	Completed EBP: A mock trial approach presentation and provided opportunities for nurses in both the inpatient areas and outpatient clinics.	Nursing education team created a mock trial using the theme "To Glove or Not" to provide examples of using the evidence to guide nursing practice.

(continues)

Exhibit 14-2 (continued)

Projected Plan to Implement and Hardwire EBP at Veterans Affairs Gulf Coast Veterans Healthcare System (VAGCHVCS): Plan of Action and Milestones

Objectives	Action Item	Action Leader/ Start Date	Completion Date	Measure of Effectiveness	Comments
Provide ongoing educational opportunities on the topic of EBP.	Integrate EBP principles into nursing grand rounds.	Employees	November 2009—15 participants	Scheduled nursing grand rounds with related EBP topic.	Jennifer White provided presentation on how to critically appraise the literature. Will plan on additional topics for nursing grand rounds.
Increase direct care/ bedside nurses' involvement in facility EBP.	Obtain approval from NCP to create a Mosby's nursing skills subcommittee that consists of at least 75% direct care nurses. This subcommittee	Employee	January 2010	Creation of NCP Mosby's nursing skills subcommittee.	January 2010 NCP approved subcommittee. This first nursing skills to be reviewed were sent to subcommittee

	is to review and revise existing and updated nursing procedures located in the VAGCVHCS.			members in February 2010. Plan to submit committee members for incentive reward per local station memorandum
Increase nursing research activity at VAGCVHCS.	Partner with university affiliate to create a nursing research committee.	Employees	Nursing research committee established at VAGCVHCS.	Initial meeting with affiliating university and psychology chief) will develop memorandum of understanding. Elicited examples of charters, SOPs, and policy from other VAMCs. One nursing research study pending

(continues)

Exhibit 14-2 *(continued)*

Projected Plan to Implement and Hardwire EBP at Veterans Affairs Gulf Coast Veterans Healthcare System (VAGCHVCS): Plan of Action and Milestones

Objectives	Action Item	Action Leader/ Start Date	Completion Date	Measure of Effectiveness	Comments
Create a formal VAGCVHCS nursing group to support and hardwire EBP within the system	1. Obtain support from advanced practice nursing committee. 2. Conduct a needs assessment. 3. The work group is to create a charter. 4. Submit charter to nursing leadership for approval.			Creation of VAGCVHCS evidence-based practice committee.	IRB review, one nursing research study completing training and preparing for IRB submission. Anticipate this will occur by January 2011.

NCP = Nursing Clinical Practice, VAMC = Veterans Affairs Medical Center.

In our project, assignments were made based on expertise, and volunteers took other assignments.

An informal discussion and needs assessment determined that the majority of nursing staff at our facility were uncomfortable with and lacked concrete knowledge about the EBP process. Without a strong foundation of EBP, it would be difficult to disseminate. Increasing knowledge of EBP for facility nursing staff was identified as our priority. Nursing education took on this challenge and created a number of training evolutions. The first education opportunity utilized a mock trial to produce a fun, nonthreatening approach to engage nursing staff. Continuing education units were obtained to encourage staff attendance. The nursing education department created and conducted a mock trial that highlighted the topic of hand washing. This subject was chosen because it impacts all nurses, regardless of specialty. Entitled "To Glove or Not," the mock trial consisted of a judge, jury, four witness, and two attorneys. Evidence related to hand hygiene and gloving was presented and examined. Postpresentation, an audience discussion was facilitated to assess the group's understanding of the best evidence. The presentation received positive feedback. Likert evaluation of the objectives revealed a 4.8 appraisal. The Likert scale assessed the achievement of the objectives from 1 to 5, with 1 being completely disagree and 5 being completely agree.

The next training evolution delved deeper into EBP, and a 1-hour continuing education unit about how to critically appraise the literature was provided. The acting nurse manager on the medical-surgical floor was a certified nurse leader (CNL) and agreed to do the presentation. We utilized nursing grand rounds as a platform to provide the information. Continuing education units were obtained and there was good staff participation.

Future nursing grand rounds are scheduled and will focus on particular areas of our facility such as palliative care and mental health. Our plan is to introduce case studies and review of literature to encourage discussion and support current practice.

Evaluation Methods

Ninety percent of assigned work was completed within the 2-week period. Ten percent did not respond. Contact with nonrespondents was attempted three times. Continued unresponsiveness resulted in removal of the nonrespondent from his or her subcommittee.

Outcomes With Impact

Recognition is paramount to ensure sustained commitment and motivation in most projects. Our hospital organization has numerous avenues to recognize exceptional contributions through both monetary and time-off means. We plan to recommend all subcommittee members who participated for a reward of 8 hours leave per procedure reviewed. We anticipate that this will create a sense of value and create excitement concerning this project. It is imperative that direct care nurses are involved in clinical practice and have a keen understanding of EBP. Nurses want autonomy in practice. This level of engagement will ensure increased professionalism in nursing practice and produce cost-efficient quality delivery of nursing care.

Project planning to incorporate EBP in a facility must be well planned, include exceptional communication, and contain clearly defined objectives and leadership endorsement. Once the nursing population achieved increased awareness of EPB, the next step was to increase involvement of direct care nursing staff. A subcommittee was established through nurse clinical practice (NCP) to review current nursing policies. Nurse managers were asked to recommend bedside nurses from each department to participate.

Our facility utilizes vendor-purchased electronic nursing skills procedure software. Each month, the vendor provides multiple updates. The nursing clinical practice committee is required to review all updates, compare them to existing policies and best practice, and apply them to our unique patient population to determine if the updates will be accepted. Through the subcommittee, nursing procedures were assigned to direct care nurses to review. Assignments were made according to area of specialty. Ambulatory care nurses were assigned to injections, surgical nurses to sterile techniques, ICU nurses to transvenous pacing, etc. Subcommittee members were partnered with a mentor and sent a letter that explained the process. A 2-week time frame to review the procedures and submit to the subcommittee chairperson was explained. Recommendations were uploaded to the NCP SharePoint site for NCP members to review and comment. Electronic comments and discussion were completed prior to the NCP meeting. Any unresolved issues were presented to the NCP by the subcommittee chairperson at the monthly meeting for assessment, discussion, and concurrence.

Initially, mass confusion ensued by all who accepted the responsibility. Even though a letter was sent to each participant outlining the procedure, the subcommittee members were unsure and overwhelmed by the initial process. We reviewed and modified the participant letter. Because we listed the mentor and nurse manager in the letter, the nurses had a contact person to walk them through the process.

References

Polit, D., & Beck, C. (2008). *Nursing research: Generating and assessing evidence for nursing practice* (8th ed.). Philadelphia: Lippincott Williams & Wilkins.

Roussel, L., Swansburg, R. C., & Swansburg, R. J. (2006). *Management and leadership for nurse administrators* (4th ed.). Sudbury, MA: Jones and Bartlett.

Staffing Methodology for Veterans Health Administration Nursing Personnel: Setup for a National Program

Alan Bernstein

Problem Statement

The purpose of this project was to develop and implement a standardized, data-driven staffing methodology for Veterans Health Administration (VHA) nursing personnel.

Gap in Knowledge Addressed by the Project

A standardized nurse staffing methodology will support a national process to systematically measure the impact of nurse staffing on patient care outcomes. Accordingly, facilities will have the necessary tools and methods to aggregate, share, and compare data with one another, ultimately leading to the creation of staffing benchmarks. This, in turn, leads to continuous quality improvement and results in the provision of increasingly effective, efficient, and high-quality health care for veterans. The expected benefits are:

- Standardized resource management tool to facilitate the development of a business case for nurse staffing budget allocation
- System-wide comparative data analysis to assist management decisions and provide for national benchmarking and comparative analysis
- Patient outcomes linked to nurse staffing levels, skill mix, and nursing hours per patient day (NHPPD) for continuous quality improvement

Team Development

Facility coordinators worked with end users to monitor, document, and provide general on-site oversight of the pilot process and facilitate communication between the staff and project manager. The facility coordinator generated status reports and briefed the project manager monthly or on an as-needed basis (e.g., training issues, process issues, issues with the staffing tools, documentation of solutions proposed and lessons learned) and provided his or her sites with updates on the status of the pilot and reports from the executive steering committee (ESC). Facility trainers worked in coordination with the facility coordinator and were responsible for the training of staff with respect to the staffing tools and methodology process in general. They were consistently available for troubleshooting to address all training issues and to document challenges encountered and proposed solutions.

Process Management

In order to be sure that we were on track with community standards and current with trends in nurse staffing, a number of meetings were held. The nature and results of those meetings follow.

- Met with nursing expert in the field of staffing and methodologies.
- Convened a staffing methodology action team to build the program.
- Convened a staffing methodology review team to critique the work of the staffing methodology action team.

- Developed and implemented a pilot of the methodology.
- Conducted focus groups and surveyed pilot participants to evaluate effectiveness of the program.
- Developed a national policy for staffing plans as well as a policy for staffing methodology for nursing personnel.
- Conducted a national survey for NHPPD for comparative analysis.
- Developed a national share point site (shared drive) for distribution of all materials.

A multiphased implementation strategy was designed to assist each site in the identification, prioritization, scheduling, and management of the pilot activities that needed to be accomplished. The phases of pilot implementation were:

- Prepilot—July to October, 2008
- Staff training—October 7–8, 2008
- Facility preparation—October 9–31, 2008
- Pilot launch—November 3, 2008 to January 31, 2009
- Closeout—February 2 to March 31, 2009

Testing of the staffing methodology workbook (instructions and supporting tools) served several purposes, which included:

1. Examination of the reliability and user friendliness of the process
2. Functionality, reliability, and accuracy of the workbooks
   a. Practice setting worksheets
   b. Replacement factor calculator
   c. NHPPD calculator
3. Test and finalize the formula/method for calculating NHPPD using decision support systems data
4. Revision and final drafting of FAQs, tutorial PowerPoint presentations, and talking points for the staffing methodology process implementation tool kit

Two teams were established for the purposes of the pilot—a national ESC and a facility pilot management team. The ESC assumed ultimate responsibility for the planning, executing, and evaluation of the pilot. The team was composed of Office of Nursing (ONS) program directors, the ONS pilot (project) manager, the national nursing executive council nursing practice transformation goal group chairperson, and ad hoc members of the staffing methodology action team. The ESC convened monthly or as needed to review progress reports from the ONS pilot manager and provide oversight to ensure adherence to objectives and timelines. The ONS pilot (project) manager served as the primary point of contact for the pilot management team and reported to the ESC. The project manager documented and summarized facility team status reports and proposed solutions to challenges encountered. The pilot management team consisted of the facility coordinator and facility trainer and convened monthly or as needed to provide periodic reports to the project manager.

Evaluation Methods

Monitoring of the process was built on the concept of continuous quality improvement. Targeted surveys commenced following the pilot closeout. The evaluation of the pilot was achieved through documentation of the following elements:

1. Functionality: The extent to which the process meets the organization's goals and objectives
2. Errors and exceptions: Documentation and analysis of process short-comings and proposed solutions
3. User satisfaction: A review of the extent to which the system meets or exceeds expectations of staff

Outcomes With Impact

The NHPPD inventory report provides comparisons between points of care–reported NHPPD and decision support systems–reported NHPPD. The report further provides baseline information about the number of direct care hours provided per patient day as well as standardization of facility nursing units across the system. This data will guide and support the development of a standardized method to determine appropriate direct care staff for nursing personnel. This will support the process to measure the impact of staff levels and staff mix on patient outcomes.

Reference

Austin, C. & Boxerman, S. (2003). *Information systems for healthcare management.* Chicago: Health Administration Press, p. 311.

RN Residency Program

Alan Bernstein and Kerrian Reynolds

Problem Statement

The purpose of this national implementation plan is to provide information and guidance for implementation of the VHA Registered Nurse (RN) Residency Program within the VHA. This plan contains activities of ONS staff, directly involved with this project, and the RN Residency Program steering committee members.

Gap in Knowledge Addressed by the Project

The RN Residency Program is designed as a 12-month developmental program that includes clinical, leadership, and professional transition elements created to assist a new graduate nurse in attaining the program objectives. The structure of the program is designed around core curriculum content based on the post-baccalaureate residency program accreditation standards of the Commission on Collegiate Nursing Education, which include:

1. Precepted clinical experiences
2. Formal mentorship
3. Resident support group meetings (clinical debriefings)
4. Monthly seminars to address various clinical practice, professional development, and leadership topics
5. Complete, multipoint resident performance/competency assessments and overall program evaluation

Team Development

At the national level, the RN Residency Program national steering committee was convened by ONS to design, implement, and oversee the activities of this project. The group is cochaired by a nurse executive and nurse educator and facilitated by an ONS program director and project manager (project team members/national steering committee). The composition of this committee consists of nursing education representatives, employee education experts, and nurse managers from various facilities across the VHA. Before implementation, the responsibilities of the group were to design and successfully launch the program. After implementation, this core group will oversee the program pilot and then continue to serve as a consultative body once the program is implemented at the national level. This group communicates via periodic (weekly or biweekly) conference calls maximizing various group communication technologies (Windows Net Meeting, Microsoft Live Meeting, etc.). Stakeholders of this program include all VHA nursing staff involved in recruiting, educating, and training new graduate RNs such as RN Residency Program coordinators, nurse preceptors/mentors, nurse managers, and nurse recruiters.

Process Management

This implementation plan is a tool for the project team to use to develop the implementation process and plan the implementation effort. This implementation plan will be updated with current information throughout the project's life cycle and provides the following information:

- Scope of implementation
- Tentative schedule for implementation from initial preparation through testing and national rollout
- Tools to be used for implementation
- Resources needed and roles/responsibilities for implementation

Evaluation Methods

Clinical flow sheets showing implementation activities will be developed at all of the VA Medical Centers that contain an ICU. It is recommended that each medical center director appoint an RN Residency Program coordinator for their site. This role is instrumental in effectively carrying out all activities related to the yearlong program. This role may be filled by an experienced nurse educator, nurse recruiter, or related nurse with experience in clinical/ nursing education and training.

Outcomes With Impact

The major outcomes of the residency program will be as follows: improved turnover/enhanced retention: improved recruitment (competition); standardized competencies of new graduate nurses among VA medical centers system-wide; succession planning; and validation of the business case for the program. Implementation of a standardized RN residency program system-wide will enhance retention and recruitment possibilities for the VHA with the new graduate nurse population.

Summary

The application of project management concepts and principles provided through the examples in this chapter give positive proof that a rigorous plan can make a difference. It is imperative that project planning become an integral component of students' clinical and field experiences. Understanding these concepts allows for transferring these newfound skills into practice setting.

INDEX

Page numbers followed by *b*, *f*, or *t* indicate boxed text, figures, or tables, respectively. Numbers followed by *exhibit* indicate exhibits.